NOW

With You

NOW

Without

ALSO BY KATHRYN LEIGH SCOTT

The Happy Hours

Last Dance at the Savoy

Jinxed

Down and Out in Beverly Heels

Dark Passages

Dark Shadows: Return to Collinwood

The Bunny Years

Dark Shadows Memories

Lobby Cards: The Classic Films

Lobby Cards: The Classic Comedies

NOW

With You

NOW

Without

My Journey
Through Life and Loss

KATHRYN
LEIGH SCOTT

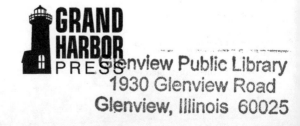

GRAND
HARBOR
PRESS

Published by Grand Harbor Press, Grand Haven, MI

www.brilliancepublishing.com

Amazon, the Amazon logo, and Grand Harbor Press are trademarks of Amazon.com, Inc., or its affiliates.

ISBN-13: 9781542046732
ISBN-10: 1542046734

Cover design by Angela Moody

Printed in the United States of America

For Geoff
and for all caregivers and their loved ones

When you arise in the morning think on what a precious privilege it is to live—to breathe—to think— to enjoy—to love!

—*Marcus Aurelius*

Contents

AUTHOR'S NOTE

I'm grateful that the neurologist who diagnosed my husband advised me to keep a daily journal, a practical suggestion I recommend to all caregivers. After my husband passed away, I drew on the journal to write a memoir, *Last Dance at the Savoy: Life, Love and Caring for Someone with Progressive Supranuclear Palsy* (2016). I also became a national volunteer spokesperson on behalf of CurePSP, a nonprofit foundation focused on neurodegenerative diseases. Speaking to caregivers and participating in support groups across the country has given me a fresh perspective. I've drawn on this, my memoir and my journal to write *Now With You, Now Without* about making the most of the time we have left with loved ones and resuming life in a world without them.

PART ONE

LIVE LIFE FULLY; DON'T WASTE A PRECIOUS
MOMENT OF IT.

Chapter One

Many years ago, an English woman with captivating charm and a steely glint in her eye told me, "Of course you're up to it, my dear. If not now, when?"

Her spirit was indomitable, and her words, spoken with cut-crystal diction, were all I needed to give me the confidence to audition for a role in a new play at one of Britain's finest repertory theatres. I got the job, and the woman I regarded as my mentor attended one of the first previews to cheer me on.

The time was the early 1970s. I was a young American actress, new to London and starting fresh, scared to death I'd made a terrible mistake leaving behind a promising theatrical and film career in New York. I'd left the freakishly successful afternoon soap *Dark Shadows* at the height of its popularity to move to London with my soon-to-be first husband. Uprooting myself hadn't been an entirely frivolous decision, but as eagerly as I embraced this new chapter in my life, I also knew I was jeopardizing a budding career doing work I loved. I signed with a wonderful new English agent, but I otherwise felt unmoored trying to navigate an unfamiliar culture I found both exhilarating and intimidating.

Soon after I arrived in London, I was introduced to Jane, a rail-thin woman with elegantly sculpted cheekbones and a fancy double-barreled last name, who I guessed had to be in her early seventies. She was delightfully eccentric, with sparkling blue eyes, a warm smile and a coiffed pouf of lavender-tinted hair. She said she was a teacher.

"Of what?" I asked.

"Everything!" she trilled in her musical voice. "Whatever you want to learn."

"Then teach me," I said impulsively, responding to an unmistakable sense that she was someone of rare talent and intellect that I wanted to get to know better.

At three o'clock the following Wednesday afternoon, I made my way to Wigmore Hall, a renowned concert venue near Marylebone High Street, where Jane had a small rehearsal studio on an upper floor that came equipped with a ballet barre and a piano. For the sum of five pounds (roughly twelve dollars back then), Jane taught me whatever she felt like teaching me that day. I rarely knew in advance if we were going to work on voice, movement, poetry, scene study or accents or discuss some aspect of British life or history, although her choice of wardrobe for the day was often a clue. Occasionally I would arrive to find her at the barre wearing a leotard, but more often she clothed her lithe figure in one of her many floaty chiffon tea dresses or stylishly tailored brocade suits.

As long as I lived in London and she was up to it, I took a weekly class with Jane that occasionally turned into a field trip, such as when she invited me to a local tearoom to teach me the customs of a proper English tea, or to a concert where she introduced me to beautifully sung German lieder. In her studio, it didn't matter that I spoke no Italian and lacked the voice to be an opera singer; I learned the arias that Jane assigned and sang them as she played the piano. I practiced various Welsh, Scottish and English accents; read poetry; did pliés at the barre and worked on improvisational scenes with her.

Beyond the Shakespearean sonnets, Puccini arias and Noël Coward plays, I learned such a lot about life from Jane. As a youngster she'd studied ballet and danced at Sadler's Wells Theatre before turning to acting both in films and on stage. She married an army officer, lived in various places abroad, raised a son and nursed her beloved husband, who had suffered severe war injuries. She'd lived a calamitous life and begun afresh many times, her grit apparent from the struggles and periods of severe hardships she'd endured. But as she would say, "One gets on with it. This is life, not a dress rehearsal."

Despite the vast difference in our ages, we were confidants. She let me know with a coquettish wink that there was romance in her life, a doctor somewhat younger than her, who shared her love of music and ballet. In turn, I confided in Jane, expressing my most personal thoughts, knowing I could trust her to respond with candor and understanding. She had always pushed the boundaries herself, embracing formidable new ventures, and urged me to stretch myself. She encouraged me to write. She challenged me to learn new skills and take on projects that seemed beyond me, always exhorting, "If not now, when?"

Beginning in 1978, I was offered roles in various productions that took me to Hollywood, which meant seeing less of Jane. However, our relationship only deepened through prolific correspondence. *Your lovely letter arrived in the afternoon post,* she'd write, *and I've taken pen in hand to respond immediately . . . such a lot to address, dear girl!*

We wrote each other so frequently that our letters formed an ongoing conversation. I'd receive six-to-eight-page letters written in her elegant script, in blue ink on fine notepaper, that I'd read over and over until her next letter arrived. Jane's insights and encouragement provided me with the support I needed in those early days in Hollywood when I was once again starting afresh. She bucked me up when I was discouraged and cheered me on when things were going well. In particular, I remember the opening sentence of her lengthy response to a question I'd posed in a previous letter: *My dear girl, we still have such a lot to work on together . . .*

Eventually, the pilot I'd filmed for a primetime CBS television series was picked up, and my stays in Los Angeles grew lengthier. By then Jane had become frail. During my visits to London, we usually spent our time together over afternoon tea sharing confidences of a more intimate nature. We were both in periods of transition, with Jane's end-of-life passage contrasting with my own burgeoning career, our trajectories seemingly worlds apart. But we shared a strong bond, unspoken but understood: we were each facing the unknown as an adventure, something new to be experienced. She was unafraid; could I show less courage?

Jane was immaculately groomed, wearing a plum velvet suit, when we met for the last time in a fusty old-world tearoom off Oxford Street that had become our favorite place to indulge in scones served warm with jam and clotted cream. I knew she was very ill, but she didn't let it dampen her spirits or curtail her remarkable appetite. She was happy I'd been signed to a television series and knew I'd be gone for some time. She was also aware that I was contemplating more personal transitions in my life, and offered counsel and encouragement.

"We come into this world alone and leave it alone; we must make peace with who we are and what we leave behind," she told me that afternoon. Her voice was soft but her tone unflinching. "We must aim high and become the best of ourselves."

I was in Los Angeles when I received a letter from her son letting me know Jane had passed away. I was heartbroken, our decade-long friendship not nearly enough time for me to fully know the woman who'd guided me through more than a few upheavals and rough patches. Over the years, I thought of all the things I wished I'd asked her, yet I had notebooks crammed with her life's lessons, including: *Live life fully; don't waste a precious moment of it.* Jane lived her own life by that dictum and impressed upon me to do the same, to make the hard decisions and move on with grace.

In the decades since our last tea together, Jane's words have come to mind many times, providing encouragement—and courage!—to handle the unexpected and take on what seemed beyond my ability to achieve. I still think of her often. Her photograph hangs on my wall as a reminder to embrace life fully.

Indeed, *If not now, when?*

Chapter Two

During our last tea together, when I confided to Jane the shifts I foresaw in my personal life, I could not have imagined they would eventually involve a man I'd met briefly many years earlier. Had Jane known Geoff, she would have found him a kindred spirit and would have loved his deep, resonant voice and roguish smile—she may even, upon first seeing him, have believed he was an actor. So I thought when, introduced to him at a press party in New York in 1968, I was struck by his magnetic presence. Tall and slim, with dark, curly hair, he looked like Clark Kent with his black-framed eyeglasses—and was a dead ringer for Superman without them. He arrived at the party in the company of writer Tom Wolfe, whose book *The Electric Kool-Aid Acid Test* I'd just read. I chatted with the two of them for a few minutes, then spent most of the evening talking with Geoff, discovering we shared many interests, including writing, traveling, traditional jazz, 1930s-era films and art deco.

Geoff wasn't an actor, although he'd hankered to study theatre arts in college, but he *had* grown up in Tinseltown with movie stars for neighbors. While doing graduate work in journalism at UCLA, winning awards for his writing, he'd designed the prototype for *Los Angeles* magazine. He launched the first issue in the summer of 1960. His template for a city-centric lifestyle magazine became hugely successful, spawning imitators across the country—including *New York* magazine, for which Tom Wolfe had just written a piece.

With the party in full swing around us, Geoff and I sat, knees touching, engrossed in our wide-ranging conversation. As captivated as I was by his Hollywood stories (he'd been an altar boy at Elizabeth Taylor's first wedding to Nicky Hilton), he was intrigued by my life as an actress on the Gothic soap *Dark Shadows*. He won me over with his ironic humor, speculating about what television's standards and practices would allow a vampire to get up to on daytime television. Long after midnight, he reluctantly said goodbye—he had an early flight back to Los Angeles—then suggested we head to a pub on the corner for an Irish coffee. He didn't want the evening to end, nor did I. But despite our mutual attraction, we were both involved in committed relationships and working on opposite coasts. Romance was off the table.

In 1971 I married Ben Martin, a photojournalist with *Time* magazine, and moved to England to live and work. In 1974 Geoff married Barbara, a lively mother of two school-age children and, coincidentally, a West Coast–based stringer with *Time*. Soon after their wedding, Barbara was diagnosed with multiple sclerosis (MS), a debilitating disease affecting the brain and spinal cord. Geoff ran *Los Angeles* magazine while nursing her; the early-onset disease never went into remission, and she passed away in 1985.

While Ben traveled the world on assignment, I began splitting my time living and working between London and Los Angeles. Home in London was a two-story cottage built in 1791, the first house built in the Sheep's Meadow of Marylebone, a stone's throw from Marble Arch and Hyde Park. In the Hollywood Hills in Los Angeles, I'd moved into a pretty little house, called *Le Provençal*, with its own storied history. Purportedly built by studio head Jack Warner for his trysts with starlets, it was said to be haunted by the mother of a thirties film star. The house must have sagged with relief when I moved in bringing no fresh notoriety, but I did convert a small pavilion in the garden into a writing room with a newfangled home computer that used floppy disks. The room also became headquarters for Pomegranate Press, a publishing company specializing in nonfiction entertainment subjects that I launched with Ben.

Unfortunately, that period also marked the collapse of my marriage, the transition I foresaw in my final few chats with Jane. Ben and I had been growing apart, but with our high regard for each other intact, we managed our separation so amicably we remained friends and continued to share our London Cottage. Jane's sage observation over tea that showing kindness and civility was the surest way to avoid an adversarial relationship saw me through this terribly painful passage.

A short time later, a *Los Angeles* magazine editor chose a coffee-table book I'd written on film art for their best Christmas gift feature and proposed interviewing me over lunch. When I arrived at the office, none other than Geoff Miller, the managing editor of the magazine, dropped by.

In that serendipitous remeeting, more than two decades after we'd first met in New York, Geoff took my hand to congratulate me—and I was once again captivated by his warmth and charm. He loved my book on classic films and reminded me we'd talked late into the night about favorite screwball comedies. I remembered our knees touching. We continued to hold hands as we chatted and walked to the elevator, not letting go until the doors began closing. Throughout my lunch with the editor, my thoughts were on Geoff. I knew I didn't want another twenty years to pass without seeing him. Late that afternoon he called to invite me for lunch the following day, and that was the beginning of our life together. On May 27, 1991, we married in Napa Valley, California.

I've condensed two decades, several lives and some of life's messiest, most unpredictable passages into a few pages, but that's the nature of memory. I recall more that was wonderful than not, including that my first husband, Ben, became close friends with Geoff and me, and the three of us shared the use of our beloved London Cottage—a home away from home and a launchpad for travel throughout Europe that none of us could bear to give up.

It's fitting that, even in the beginning, my relationship with Geoff spanned two coasts. An editor once waggishly remarked that Geoff "created a city magazine that tells you how to get out of town!"—a reference to the innovative *Weekend Guide*, annual *Restaurant Guide* and all the "Best" lists, most involving travel features, that he created and which were emulated by city magazines everywhere.

Our shared passion for travel quickly became an intoxicating ingredient in our courtship, one that never flagged throughout our lives together. Geoff's ventures abroad had been far more limited than mine, and he was envious that I'd toured Europe on my own as a teenager and had the opportunity to live and work in Paris and London. He wanted to make up for lost time, especially the magazine's frenetic start-up years when he was tethered to a demanding workload.

Constant throughout our marriage was the anticipation of travel: calendars marked, tickets in hand, always preparing to go somewhere. At first there was the romance of introducing each other to places we'd discovered on our own and wanted to share, then the adventure of discovering new destinations we could explore together. We returned to favorite spots again and again, and there was romance in that, too: booking the same room in a hotel or hiking familiar paths that held significance for us.

During our early years together, I guest starred in episodes of numerous television series, often filming in distant locations. When I filmed in Hawaii, London and various stateside locales, Geoff joined me for long weekends. In turn, I would meet him in New York or San Francisco for a few days at the tail ends of his business trips. On one occasion, I got a magazine assignment to write about the reopening of the Dorchester hotel in London. Geoff was already booked on the press junket on behalf of *Los Angeles* magazine, so we traveled together, enjoying a round-trip flight on the Concorde and a glittery five-day getaway.

A travel magazine assigned me to write a piece about the *Hurtigruten*, the Norwegian ships plying regular daily routes on the western coast from the southern city of Bergen to Kirkenes, a northern village near the Finnish and Russian borders. Since the trip in 1994 coincided with Geoff's retirement from *Los Angeles* magazine and my mother's eightieth birthday, both joined me on our ten-day excursion. The assignment provided the perfect opportunity to immerse Geoff in my heritage (my father and both sets of grandparents were Norwegian immigrants) and the splendors of a country where I'd lived as a child and often visited as an adult. Every few hours we'd pull into another port along the route, and as mail and freight were loaded and new passengers boarded, we would disembark for a stroll around town. While my mother and I indulged in *rømmegrøt* and *smørrebrød* (cream pudding and open-faced sandwiches), Geoff would tease us about "your people" coming up with so many resourceful ways to serve Jell-O and herring, though fortunately not in combination.

On that memorable trip, we stayed with my mother's cousins in the Valdres region and visited my father's village in Romsdal, where our family lived when I was a toddler. By the light of the midnight sun, we joined some twenty cousins for an evening of revelry on the island in the fjord below my father's former farm.

But as much as he enjoyed foreign travel, nothing appealed to Geoff more than plotting the route for a magical road trip close to home. He'd grown up in California and was ardent about the beauty of its mountains, beaches, forests, deserts, vineyards and glorious rugged coastline. Our annual Thanksgiving trip was a leisurely drive up Highway One along the coast through Carmel and Big Sur to Mendocino. Geoff took pleasure in consulting his annotated files of brochures, guidebooks and maps in search of a remote gem of natural beauty or an obscure historical site to explore. He was always on the lookout for a new restaurant, a local music festival or an art event to feature in *Los Angeles* magazine.

In 2007, sixteen years into our marriage, life was sweet. Geoff had been retired from the magazine for thirteen years but was doing consulting work for a New York–based publishing company. I was busy acting and writing.

We frequently stayed in the London Cottage, using it as a hub for spontaneous jaunts to Paris, Dublin, Prague, Saint Petersburg—wherever we could get a last-minute budget flight on EasyJet or Ryanair. For our sixteenth wedding anniversary in May, we'd planned a side trip to Italy—a mix of business and pleasure, since I'd been invited to attend STICCON, the Italian *Star Trek* convention, as a celebrity guest at the annual meeting of Trekkies. I'd portrayed Nuria in the fan-favorite "Who Watches the Watchers" episode of *Star Trek: The Next Generation.*

Entranced by the view of the Adriatic from the balcony of our seaside hotel room, we opted to stroll on the Bellaria beach instead of napping after our journey from London. The picturesque seashore, bedecked with colorful cabanas and neat rows of old-fashioned canvas chairs, had the charm of a vintage prewar postcard. Barefoot and clad in T-shirts and bathing suits, we giddily headed for the shimmering shoreline. With the sun hot on our shoulders, we waded into the chill surf toward a weathered pier, pale in the distance. I was the first to reach it, and turned back to warn Geoff to duck under the low beam. He did, but not quickly enough; he struck his head, falling backward into the water.

With blood gushing from his head wound, we were raced to the town's infirmary where Geoff was given a tetanus shot and had his wound stitched up. I smiled encouragingly, but I was shaken by the sight of him lying on a gurney, his face bloodstained. The mishap could be blamed on travel fatigue, the sun's glare, a stumble or misjudgment, but I felt a deep sense of disquiet at the realization that incidents like this had become more frequent.

A year earlier, in the jostling rush-hour crowd in the London Underground, Geoff had lost his balance and fallen backward down the escalator, injuring his head and shoulder. Paramedics transported us to a local hospital, where he was stitched up and bandaged. While we blamed the accident on rambunctious schoolchildren, I felt responsible for not holding his arm to keep him steady—why hadn't I paid closer attention to prevent the accident from occurring? I realized I'd begun unconsciously taking on that role wherever we went. My natural reaction was to hold a door open, look out for cracks in the pavement and avoid slippery grass, all without being aware of how protective I had become.

Unfortunately there were lapses when I wasn't in a position to hold his arm. On one occasion, Geoff impulsively climbed to the top deck of a London bus, missed a step and tumbled down the steep stairs. The other passengers were horrified to see him insist on climbing back up the stairs, but Geoff grinned and claimed he wasn't injured. Little pleased him more than sitting in the coveted front seats on the top deck. He laughed off my concern, claiming he'd been clumsy and would be more careful.

I took stock of Geoff's frequent accidents, vowing to be more careful as we negotiated cobbled streets, steep stairs and various other hazards on our trip. Booked into a fancy Venice hotel suite to celebrate our wedding anniversary, I glanced at the slippery sides of the deep marble bathtub, with no grip bars on the walls, and saw disaster looming. We showered instead. On our flight back to London, wearing an Italian school cap to cover the stitches in his head, Geoff was already looking forward to our next trip.

Geoff laughed off any attempts on my part to dissuade him from taking trips, pointing out that these accidents could happen at home just as easily—and they did. I'd already removed throw rugs and whatever obstacles in our house might cause him to slip or stumble, but falls still occurred. The solution wasn't for us to stay home, but for me to be even more vigilant. Undeterred by mishaps along the way, Geoff just wanted to keep traveling.

Chapter Three

It wasn't Geoff's accident that curtailed our stay in Europe that spring, but rather an urgent call from Minneapolis. I flew directly there from London to care for my mother, who had been diagnosed with an advanced stage of lymphoma and, at age ninety-two, opted for palliative care. While I stayed in Minneapolis, Geoff remained in Los Angeles.

My mother needed me, and I wanted the precious time with her, but I was uneasy about Geoff living on his own, particularly as the head wound he'd suffered in Italy was still healing. His too-frequent stumbles and falls concerned me. His gait seemed plodding and he "plopped" when he sat down. He tired easily. His speech was slow, his voice some-times faint. Too often things slipped from his hands and broke. He no longer seemed to care about his personal appearance and was often edgy and irritable. He would attribute any lapses to "just growing older" and jokingly say, "consider the alternative." I'd laugh, but doubted these changes in behavior were due solely to aging.

Meanwhile, my mother's ninety-third birthday was coming up, and she delegated the arrangements for her party to me. Although the kitchen in her senior-living apartment was her domain, she was too weak to prepare the chicken salad and walnut-banana bread herself, and hovered at my elbow supervising. She also wanted to make *kransekake*, an elaborate Norwegian wedding cake, for which she was renowned.

Unable to do it herself, she watched as I grated two pounds of blanched almonds a handful at a time, whisked egg whites and sifted confectioners' sugar, all to her exacting specifications. As a youngster, I'd helped her with the labor-intensive process of hand-rolling fifteen circles of almond dough into special baking tins, but we both knew this would be my last opportunity to make a *kransekake* under my mother's tutelage. The *kransekake*, decorated with icing and miniature Norwegian flags, was perfection. The afternoon spent with my mother making it is a memory I will always treasure.

My mom passed away only six weeks after her diagnosis. Geoff joined me for the funeral, but when we returned home to Los Angeles, I could tell he had experienced considerable difficulty living on his own during my absence. His desk was piled high with unopened mail. Friends who had taken him to dinner reported that he'd seemed unsteady, a bit disoriented. I knew he'd fallen because I could see his bruises. Back on home turf, gestures that had simply seemed idiosyncratic, such as the odd way he tried to adjust his eyeglasses when he wasn't wearing any, now struck me as worrying. He would awkwardly attempt to open a wine bottle with one hand instead of two and struggled to do anything that required coordinating his hands. I'd fallen into the habit of resting my thumb against the base of his wineglass so that he wouldn't tip it over when he reached for it. He would tap surfaces before setting something down, a sign, I only later came to learn, of his inability to judge depth and distance.

Geoff thrived on being around other people, and we had an active social life, frequently entertaining at home. An affable host, he made everyone feel welcome, drawing each guest into dinner table conversation that was lively and fun. Geoff's great gift was tossing off zingers that caught everyone by surprise, but I noticed he now seemed lethargic, his energy spent soon after guests arrived. He'd lapse into silence at the dinner table, sitting with his elbow propped on the table, his hand supporting his head, not looking up from his plate. He ate with one hand, awkwardly shoveling food to his mouth. His eyelids would droop, and he'd give the appearance of being bored or falling asleep. When I nudged him, he'd look at me in astonishment, unaware that he'd been eating with his eyes closed.

Baffled by his conduct but trying to cover for his behavior in front of guests, I would make excuses for his drowsiness, citing sleeplessness the night before, when in fact he slept long hours and took afternoon naps. Aside from the sluggishness, I couldn't understand his uncharacteristic disregard for table manners. He would clutch a wineglass, seemingly unwilling or unable to set it back on the table. He'd saw at food with a fork instead of using a knife, and take bites that were too large and choke—then cough without covering his mouth. My continual reminders infuriated him, and he'd accuse me of berating him with a laundry list of faults. I was confounded that he could be so oblivious to what I considered rude behavior. After an evening out among friends, we'd argue or ride in silence on the way home, both of us perplexed by changes that were souring our relationship.

"You never used to complain," he'd tell me. "Now everything I do is wrong."

"But if you don't set your wineglass down, it looks like you want it refilled."

"Maybe I do."

"Not when it's already filled and you're spilling it!"

On our way out for the day, I'd notice his pants were sagging because he wasn't wearing a belt. "Why didn't you just ask me to put your belt through the loops?"

"I didn't want to bother you."

"Bother me! Better that than your pants falling down."

I tried not to complain and instead attempted to work around his moodiness and bouts of listlessness. I cut back on our social life and declined invitations that I judged too dotted with pitfalls or stressful. When I saw him struggling to open a jar or close a drawer, I'd jump in to help, which would often annoy him. But if I failed to notice he needed assistance with buttons and zippers, his temper would flare. The simplest tasks, such as opening mail or buttering toast, seemed beyond his capability. I tried to be as unobtrusive as I could in smoothing the way for him, but somehow it was always my fault if something spilled or was broken. Tempers ignited at any show of exasperation from either of us, and we'd say hurtful things neither of us meant.

It was hard to remember the carefree, easygoing relationship we'd once had, when we saw eye-to-eye and could playfully chide each other without it leading to a squabble. Our daily life had become a battle-ground over mundane issues, resulting in spiteful accusations, frustration and anger that no amount of cautious treading could reduce. Meanwhile, the adjustments I made to avoid conflict had the effect of eliminating a lot of the activities and simple pleasures we'd once enjoyed together. I was walking on eggshells, and matters seemed to grow only worse. I didn't know what to do.

The most dramatic indication of Geoff's growing impairment took place while I was in Minneapolis caring for my mother, but I didn't learn about it until months later—Geoff had kept it from me because, he said, he didn't want to "bother" me. Those words had become a common refrain and invariably portended a problem or mishap. This one came to light when an agent from our insurance company arrived at our house to discuss a claim over a vehicular incident that had been designated a felony hit-and-run.

Geoff had been charged with hitting a young jogger and leaving the scene. According to Geoff, the jogger dodged traffic and ran into his car just after the traffic light changed and he released the brake. Bracing her hands against the hood of the car, she'd leaped back just as the car rolled forward. However, from the perspective of a school-bus driver farther back from the light, it appeared that Geoff had struck the woman with his car and taken off. The bus driver was unaware that once Geoff was able to safely turn around, he went back to speak with the woman. She had resumed her jog and told him she was fine. But the bus driver had recorded Geoff's license-plate number and called the police. Complicating the situation, the jogger later told her boyfriend what had happened, and he insisted she visit an emergency room.

I believed Geoff's version of the event, but I also believed the jogger, who gave a deposition stating that he seemed "befuddled" and "not in control" when they spoke. Her statement and that of the bus driver were damning. However, in view of Geoff's unblemished driving record, evidence that he hadn't fled the scene, and the jogger's lack of injuries, the charge was reduced to a misdemeanor, but would still require a court date.

I knew appearances counted, so on the day of the hearing I made sure Geoff looked his best in a suit and tie. While most defendants were dressed in "casual Friday" attire, largely shorts and T-shirts, I hoped Geoff would look businesslike and responsible. However, I was astonished at how slumped and shrunken he appeared in the suit he'd last worn for my mother's funeral only months earlier. When he approached the bench with the attorney, he shuffled and appeared vague about his whereabouts—essentially *befuddled*. The judge spent little time questioning Geoff before suspending his driver's license, levying a fine and assigning him to community service.

I left Geoff waiting in line for his community service assignment while I went off to pay the fine and take care of other court matters. When I returned, Geoff, pale and anxious, was seated on a bench. He told me he'd lost his footing on the slick marble floor. One of the men who'd helped him to his feet told me in broken English that I needed to tell the clerk assigning road-maintenance work that my husband wasn't up to it.

Geoff was instead assigned to an HIV/AIDS food-distribution center, where he would work an eight-hour shift in a warehouse sorting food donations. The following Monday morning, we set out on the hour-long drive to the facility, Geoff making light of the fact that he hadn't been given a luminescent orange vest and assigned to clearing highway trash. But I knew he was concerned about being able to handle a full day's work lifting crates and stocking shelves. When we arrived, I volunteered to work with him in the warehouse, but my offer was declined. I left my card with the supervisor, telling him to please call me if anything happened to my husband.

I spent an anxious day concerned about his safety, worried that he would fall or injure himself. When I returned to pick him up, I found Geoff in the main building, reassigned to the client distribution counter where he was filling brown paper bags with donations. Unable to coordinate his hands, he was ripping the bags and dropping cans and jars on the floor, while impatient clients complained loudly about his inefficiency. Geoff was clearly frustrated and embarrassed, especially that I was there witnessing his humiliation. On our drive home, he was tight-lipped and moody, but told me to please pack an extra sandwich for him because he'd been given a two-hour lunch break.

Without complaint, Geoff continued to work five days a week for five weeks to fulfill his community-service commitment, most often sitting at a desk and serving as a greeter as clients arrived. He was happiest when he was offered weekend work at various grocery stores, where he collected food donations from shoppers. When he finished his shift, we'd fill a bag of our own to donate. On the way home one Saturday, he talked about some of the people he'd chatted with who had dropped off groceries, weeping when he told me that many of them were afflicted with AIDS themselves.

I knew Geoff was profoundly touched by his community-service experience, but spontaneous weeping had become an almost daily occurrence. His emotions overwhelmed him, and song lyrics, in particular, moved him to tears. His responses seemed heartfelt and genuine—but these tearful bouts were so frequent that I found them unsettling. The tenderness I felt for my husband made me reluctant to perceive his emotions as unwarranted, but I secretly wondered if he was experiencing minor strokes, which could account for his tendency to weep. We'd reached a tipping point, and I could no longer overlook what was happening.

Chapter Four

Geoff's "hit-and-run" incident was a wakeup call that forced me to confront the significant physical deterioration that had accelerated over a matter of months, including his slow, sometimes slurring speech and his cramped, almost illegible handwriting. It seemed to me that much of his inappropriate behavior emanated from physical struggles, most of it related to mobility and balance difficulties.

I was relieved his driver's license had been suspended, having been aware for some time that he wasn't the skilled, careful driver he'd once been. He was erratic, driving too slowly, stopping abruptly and tapping his foot on the accelerator as though keeping time to music. He'd wait at a stop sign an inordinate amount of time or, worse, barrel through without stopping at all. He rarely looked to the left or right. But I observed some of those same patterns of movement when he walked around the house, sometimes tapping his foot several times before taking a step or stopping in the middle of the room for no apparent reason.

Geoff was due for an annual physical with his longtime primary care physician, a jovial man with whom he had an easygoing relationship. Since Geoff couldn't drive, it was a rare opportunity for me to accompany him to the appointment. I suspected that, on his own during the exam, he would fail to mention his frequent falls and other issues, preferring to keep what he would consider minor physical annoyances to himself. Keeping a tight lid, he liked to jest, is the nature of the "guy universe." Geoff reluctantly allowed me to join him in the examining room, but only on condition that I listen and observe, not bring up a host of "faults and complaints."

I was as good as my word and said nothing, but the doctor picked up on some of the odd behavior that concerned me. In a simple balance test, Geoff was unable to stand on one foot. He had difficulty focusing his gaze. Not only couldn't he coordinate his hands to clap, but one hand made involuntary waving movements when he attempted to salute. The doctor's initial suspicion was a form of Parkinson's disease, even though Geoff had no tremors or other hallmarks of the disorder.

We followed through on appointments for other tests, including an MRI, but they revealed no strokes, tumors or inner ear problems, and nothing related to the head injury in Italy. Geoff was relieved, satisfied that whatever physical ailments he had were age related. He did not want to see any more doctors. I was anxious, convinced that he had an undiagnosed malady that should be treated.

In hindsight, I'm certain Geoff suspected he had some form of neurological impairment but preferred not to deal with it. He'd never forgotten the callous treatment by the doctor who first diagnosed Barbara with MS and told her, "Come back and see me in a year or so, but there's not much we can do for you." Indeed, there was no treatment available, and her decline was steady and rapid. In his "guy universe," if there was no cure for what ailed him, why bother?

Geoff just wanted to hit the road and keep going, but without a driver's license, he had to depend on me to get out, and that created even more tension. He did not want friends to know he couldn't drive, so we invented excuses to explain why I was dropping him off for lunch and picking him up. So he wasn't left housebound, I invited him on my rounds of errands and grocery shopping. Afterward I'd drive to the beach for lunch or stop at a newsstand so he could peruse magazine racks, one of his favorite pastimes.

Becoming a one-car household represented a major adjustment for both of us that involved more than just a vehicle. Neither of us had bargained on this turn of events; he didn't care to be dependent on me for transportation any more than I relished being his chauffeur, but that wasn't going to change. As difficult as it had been to handle the role reversal when I became my mother's caregiver, it was far more consequential when it happened with my husband. Geoff and I enjoyed being together, but now our constant companionship became an inescapable necessity. He resented his loss of freedom, but so did I. He had to accept his reliance on me; in turn, I had to show grace and tact in being available, or we would strain the delicate balance of our marital relationship. It was not easy.

One afternoon, Geoff announced that he'd called the DMV for an appointment to take the driving test that could reinstate his license. My heart sank at the prospect of having him back behind the wheel, but I drove him to the testing center at the appointed time. He passed the written exam without difficulty, unsurprising since Geoff had introduced to *Los Angeles* magazine the answers to the DMV driving test and a map of shortcuts to avoid traffic—two of its most popular features.

Prior to the road test, he practiced driving in the DMV parking lot, bewilderment clouding his face as he tried and failed to execute the maneuvers necessary to pass. Weeks later, after a morning of intense practice, he was able to pass the road test on his second try. He took a moment to enjoy his victory, then without a word handed me his car keys. Later that day we arranged to sell his car and remove his name from our automobile insurance, which had skyrocketed after his accident.

❖ ❖ ❖

Geoff's handling of the driving test revealed that even as he was rapidly losing control of his body, he was not going to relinquish the power to make his own decisions. As agonizing as it was to see him in such a quandary, I had to respect his independence. But becoming a one-car household was dissatisfying for both of us. Geoff found pleasure in driving; I drive to get somewhere as expediently as possible. Out of the corner of my eye, I observed Geoff's foot working phantom pedals on the passenger side and grimacing when I took a route he didn't favor. I chafed at always being behind the wheel, but we tried to make the best of an unhappy situation that depended on compromise and coordinated schedules.

I was both literally and figuratively in the driver's seat in so many situations that I tried to give Geoff leeway whenever I could. Despite clear signs of a movement disorder, I backed off of pushing him to have more tests and let him take the lead—which he eventually did by suggesting we make an appointment with a neurologist.

Our first appointment was with an elderly doctor in New York who specialized in treating patients with Parkinson's disease. He and Geoff hit it off immediately over a shared love of jazz. During a lively chat about favorite bands from the swing era, I realized that the doctor was using their discussion to assess Geoff's speech and cognitive faculties. Later, after a physical exam, he determined that Geoff had an unspecified movement disorder that required further evaluation. He prescribed various drugs off-label on the chance Geoff might benefit from a side effect. At the same time, he suggested I keep a daily journal to track the progression of his disease. Perhaps it was due to the doctor's genial manner, but we left his office feeling light hearted about the tentative diagnosis.

"At least it's not Parkinson's," Geoff said. "How bad can this be?"

Our next stop was the Mayo Clinic in Rochester, Minnesota, followed by the NewYork-Presbyterian/Columbia University Medical Center and finally the UCLA Department of Neurology in Los Angeles, where Geoff was officially diagnosed with progressive supranuclear palsy (PSP), a prime-of-life neurological disorder in the same family as Alzheimer's disease, Parkinson's disease, corticobasal degeneration (CBD), multiple system atrophy (MSA) and Lewy body dementia, the brain disease that afflicted actor Robin Williams. PSP, diagnosed in both actor Dudley Moore and billionaire financier Richard Rainwater, afflicts roughly twenty thousand Americans, about the same number that are diagnosed with Amyotrophic lateral sclerosis (ALS, widely known as Lou Gehrig's disease). To marked degrees, Geoff had long been exhibiting several hallmarks of the condition: frequent falls backward, a lurching gait and an inability to focus and shift his gaze.

By the time of his diagnosis, my husband, who had spent his career writing and editing, had difficulty holding a pencil or turning the page of a newspaper. Yet if we'd had a diagnosis sooner, there was nothing we could have done about it except try to keep him safe from falls and injuries. There is no treatment or cure for the disorder.

Initially, denial had been Geoff's way of coping with the baffling physical and emotional changes he was experiencing. If friends noticed his shuffling gait, slurred speech or difficulty putting on a jacket, Geoff had been adamant that I not acknowledge any health concerns. He didn't want people to treat him differently or constantly ask how he was doing. It was not in his nature to ever talk about himself or his feelings, physical or emotional. So I complied, brushing off concerns and making excuses ("he tripped on the rug"; "it's just arthritis"). But was it really better for people to think his slurred speech was caused by a drink too many or that I was turning a blind eye by not insisting that Geoff see a doctor?

As devastating as the diagnosis was, there was some relief in finally having an answer—a reaction, it turns out, that is not unusual among patients who undergo seemingly endless examinations before learning the cause of their symptoms. At least we could put a name to the ailment and figure out how to cope with its relentless, insidious progression.

And with a clear diagnosis, Geoff was open to letting people know he had PSP. At least he didn't have Parkinson's, he joked, and no one would bother figuring out what progressive supranuclear palsy was.

It was a benign form of denial that worked for Geoff and allowed me to reassure friends and family that my husband was all right, he *just* had PSP.

We determined to live our lives with as little disruption as possible. Geoff cheerfully noted he was lucky as diseases go; he suffered no pain or discomfort. As he told me, "Things could be worse."

Outwardly I embraced Geoff's upbeat attitude, but inwardly I was mourning a life together that I treasured and didn't want to lose. It seemed so improbable that we should have met—twice! I looked upon our story, the once-upon-a-time chance encounter in New York that serendipitously turned into happily-ever-after twenty years later, as a fairy tale come true. I didn't want the story to end. I couldn't imagine a time when I could no longer experience a thump of joy when Geoff walked into a room; the very thought of it filled me with dread.

My response before the diagnosis had been to deal with Geoff's behavioral changes by pulling back from our social life and other activities we'd enjoyed. Now that I knew the cause and could prepare for the inevitable progression of his disease, we couldn't waste time staying home and playing it safe, denying ourselves the pleasure of exploring the world.

I remembered Jane's ready answer whenever I expressed doubt or trepidation: "This is life, my girl. Make the most of it." It was advice that would serve me well in dealing with this passage, too. Geoff and I still had a life together, and we needed to find ways to make the most of every precious minute. The obvious answer was travel; nothing cheered Geoff more than planning a trip. Travel also meant looking ahead, anticipating new horizons and experiences, the ideal antidote to a grim diagnosis. We'd make the most of every second we had left.

I took a cue from my good friend Gretchen, a biographer and mother of three, who lives in Thief River Falls, Minnesota. Her husband and college sweetheart, Gene, a banker, had been diagnosed with Parkinson's disease some years earlier, but they hadn't let his diminishing mobility keep them from traveling. The two had even stayed with friends in our handicap-challenging London Cottage during a trip touring England. Knowing that as Gene became more symptomatic, mobility issues would curtail travel to some of the more remote, primitive destinations, they embarked on their most adventurous trips while he was up to the rigors. One of their first trips was a three-week tour of China. On another trip, Gene was so eager to explore that he'd forget he needed a walker and leave it behind for Gretchen to locate later.

The two set an example that inspired us. Knowing a trip was on the horizon would give Geoff incentive, sustaining him when it was tempting to give up. "We just don't let anything stop us," Gretchen said simply, "and I'm so glad now that we traveled the world when we could."

Geoff had always packed his own suitcase, but I took over when he began choosing unsuitable clothing and forgetting items he needed—swim trunks were not necessary in New York in January, while the dress slacks that went with his jacket were. Steadily, I assumed more responsibility when we traveled: handling the luggage for both of us when even pulling a wheeled suitcase became difficult for him, making sure I was in possession of the tickets and passports for both of us—this after a mad dash back home to retrieve them before a flight to London. I tried to take on these duties without Geoff becoming overtly aware of it; I didn't want to diminish his sense of being in charge of himself or make him feel that he was becoming a burden. My focus was entirely on making each journey pleasurable for both of us.

Our first trip was a Mediterranean cruise, and it was a boost we both needed. I bought rubber-soled walking shoes, Dockers with elastic waistbands and a fleece pullover to supplement Geoff's preferred travel attire: blue jeans, safari jackets and loafers. I also packed cotton sweaters and pullover shirts so he could dress himself with a minimum of struggle.

The ship was modest in size, not one of the multideck, crowded "floating cities" that would have overwhelmed us. In the mornings, after most other passengers disembarked for day trips, we slowly made our way onto the dock and strolled along the pier, taking a taxi to any place we couldn't reach on foot. I was delighted he managed the strenuous climbs in Taormina and Amalfi. We walked for hours, not returning to our ship until late afternoon.

The bracing sea air and spectacular, ever-changing scenery energized Geoff. I held his arm, mindful of cobbled streets, but he had no difficulty handling the steep, narrow passages in the hilltop village of Santorini. His gait seemed to improve, and we enjoyed our leisurely stroll through the winding streets of Rhodes, where we each bought a leather jacket. We knew exploring the Parthenon in Athens, Greece, and the ancient ruins near Kusadasi, Turkey, would be physically demanding, but we managed both without mishap. We took everything at our own pace, seeing as much as we could manage and indulging ourselves with plenty of rest stops along the way.

Aside from targeting all the customary tourist sites, Geoff showed off his uncanny gift for ferreting out off-beat cafés and hole-in-the-wall clubs where we could drink an aperitif while listening to a combo playing ethnic music we were unlikely to hear anywhere else. In Istanbul, we visited the markets on our own, threading our way through crowded stalls and stopping in coffee bars to sample pastries. Thanks to handrails and other safety features aboard ship, Geoff could easily maneuver around decks and corridors on his own and enjoy the solitude of sitting by himself in a deck chair.

The trip was such a success that I thought keeping Geoff on the move was the answer. A month after our return from the cruise, we cashed in more miles to spend Christmas in our New York apartment and New Year's in the London Cottage. Geoff was eager to go and seemed up to the challenge of holiday travel. Despite crowded flights and a weather delay, he was happier and more content than he'd been in a long time. His general health had markedly improved. His voice was stronger, and his speech wasn't slurred. He joined in conversation, laughing and telling stories. He had fewer bouts of moodiness, and angry outbursts were rare.

Still, I didn't want to entice the hubris dragon with overconfidence. Geoff was managing very well, but I still kept a close watch wherever we went. We took buses and subways and long walks, but I always kept a firm grip on his arm, especially on stairways and escalators. I figured out how to plant my feet and use leverage to help him sit down and stand up. We showered together as a matter of course, and I made sure he was hanging on to the faucets while I bathed him. We didn't take chances.

I did what couples generally do for each other—I accommodated, picked up the slack, pitched in and instinctively did what was necessary to keep him safe, happy and comfortable. To the world at large observing us holding hands, arms entwined, we must have looked like the happiest, most loving couple in the universe. We were inseparable, but there were plenty of diversions—perhaps all the therapy he needed was a combination of stimulating activity, exercise and companionship. Yes, travel was the antidote!

Chapter Five

As much as travel reinvigorated our marriage and kept us from focusing on the inevitable, it wasn't all moonlight and romance. Invariably we had balky interludes, which were more difficult to handle when they occurred in public. When I couldn't soothe, cajole or distract Geoff, I'd wait it out while trying to control my own emotions. He picked up on my reactions quickly, becoming even more temperamental if he saw me cry or look anxious.

My best defense was to be prepared for situations when he'd become frustrated or overwhelmed. With that in mind, I planned carefully for our trip to London, beginning with finding good-quality sweatpants with a fly front that would make using the cramped aircraft toilets easier. The Nike pants with zippered pockets were so well cut and comfortable that he didn't mind not wearing his favorite blue jeans, which required a belt that had to be removed for TSA screening. As long as I didn't separate him from his beloved safari jacket, with all its buttons and over-stuffed pockets, he was content to let me dictate his travel attire. But however well I planned ahead, I spent a sleepless night before our flight imagining every sort of disastrous scenario. I wrote a checklist in my journal: Seat Geoff on walker; remove shoes and jacket; place in bins; send Geoff through the metal detector with boarding pass in hand; fold walker; place on conveyor belt with laptop, handbag and small roller bag; race through metal detector; retrieve Geoff; clothe him; check nothing has been left behind and head for the gate. Whew.

What I hadn't counted on was the metal tab on the fly front tripping the security alarm—why hadn't I thought of that? Geoff handled the additional screening well, but I was a nervous wreck watching him tottering in his stocking feet waiting for a security guard to run a wand over his body. I knew the TSA rules didn't allow me to assist Geoff, but I was deeply concerned he would fall and injure himself.

While Geoff remained calmer than I did during the security check, I was anxious about the six-hour flight ahead of us. As my husband began to require more assistance, he wasn't always willing, or even able, to cooperate—impulsive behavior, sudden rigidity and an inability to control erratic movement are conditions associated with many neurological conditions, and they appear unexpectedly. He couldn't stop himself from lurching, or slipping out of a chair, or reaching for things that fell out of his hands and broke or spilled. I tried to prepare us for any eventuality while taking into account that Geoff wanted to remain as self-reliant as possible and not have me hovering all the time.

A rat wheel of possible catastrophes spun in my head, including Geoff falling or getting stuck in the airplane lavatory. Almost anything could spark a swift change in mood, causing him to become agitated or angry. What could I do to quiet him down if he began shouting or became abusive?

Such an incident had occurred midflight on a previous trip when a passenger walking up the aisle suddenly lurched against Geoff, causing him to spill a cup of water. Geoff was enraged the man didn't stop to apologize and shouted, his voice a harsh bark. He reached out to grab the man but was restrained by the seat belt. Fortunately a quick-witted passenger seated across the aisle took Geoff's hand and spoke softly to him before the incident could escalate. I couldn't hear what the man said, but he managed to calm Geoff, even getting him to nod and smile. A stranger had accomplished what I could not have in that moment.

I felt positively celebratory when a London taxi deposited us at the door to the Cottage and Ben was waiting for us with chilled wine, a glowing fireplace and our bed turned down. I didn't set out to cultivate two husbands (nor am I advocating it), but there were occasions when I appreciated that mine had become good friends, particularly when our visits to the Cottage overlapped.

For all its vintage charm, the Cottage had a steep, curving staircase and small upstairs bedrooms that were hazards for Geoff. Of particular concern was the deep, old-fashioned bathtub with its primitive shower arrangement. We joked that the plumbing was ancient Etruscan, but the reality of using an antiquated pull-chain toilet was a struggle for him. As much as he loved the Cottage and its proximity to Hyde Park, the high brass bed and low couch and armchairs fitted with soft cushions were not designed for his comfort or ease. Fortunately Ben could give me a hand helping him get to his feet and climb the stairs—and most helpful, engaging him in "guy" conversation that warded off moodiness.

How does one manage without two husbands? I could only hope they wouldn't conduct any private "can't-live-with-her, can't-live-without-her" chats while I was out of the room.

In the year after Geoff's diagnosis, we'd followed through on our pact to stay on the move, traveling as much as we were able, but we also needed to remain on top of his medical condition. When we returned to New York, I accompanied Geoff to a follow-up appointment with the elderly neurologist who had first diagnosed his condition. The affable doctor, who struck me from our first meeting as wise and instinctive, segued from a poignant story about hapless swing-era musicians on the road to suggesting we give practical thought to financial planning and health directives.

Thanks to the doctor's offhand, but very pointed, suggestion, we arranged a meeting with an estate planner. Geoff, who had a keen business sense, readily shared information about financial matters with me, as I did with him, but neither of us had felt comfortable broaching the topic of realistic end-of-life issues. Before Geoff became ill we didn't think about it; after his diagnosis, a conversation about death and dying felt too ominous to bring up. We'd both put it off. Yet I felt such huge relief knowing that when an emergency arose, I would have not only a power-of-attorney document, but a clear sense of how to fulfill Geoff's wishes. My mother, who was more open with her feelings, had been matter-of-fact and specific about how she wanted things handled in her last days, sparing the family from having to make hard decisions in a time of grief.

The meeting in an attorney's office provided us with the forum and structure to discuss legal matters, but after our session those talks resulted in greater openness between us about various other end-of-life issues we might not have thought to bring up. I would otherwise not have known Geoff's preference for burial, rather than cremation—nor would he have been aware I preferred the opposite.

The importance of our meeting with an estate planner was brought home to us on a weekend visit with close friends in Connecticut. Hannah, an artist and my former roommate, and Joel, a well-known magazine photographer, had a gift for finding wonderful, derelict old properties to renovate. Their rambling shoreline house, with sweeping views of Long Island Sound, was no exception. With their two sons grown, they'd turned the gabled main house, with its charming veranda, into a bed-and-breakfast, decamping to Hannah's adjacent two-story artist's studio when all the rooms were booked.

Their life was idyllic until Joel, a fit, otherwise healthy nonsmoker, was diagnosed with lung cancer. Just as Geoff had, Joel chose denial in dealing with his illness, even as he began rigorous chemo treatments. Although he had once published a manual on estate planning, Joel was unwilling to address his own health directives and end-of-life choices.

Hannah couldn't persuade him to deal with these matters, even though he had stage-four cancer and knew what was inevitable. My friend's wrenching dilemma made me that much more grateful that Geoff's doctor had opened the door for our own end-of-life discussion.

Even once I began doing all the driving on our road trips, Geoff still took charge of planning our route, mixing favorite stops with new discoveries. And he was not going to let inconvenience get in the way of his travel enjoyment. Because of his experiences caring for Barbara, it was Geoff who first suggested it was time to request handicap-equipped rooms whenever possible. "Handicap rooms didn't exist when I took Barbara on these trips," he said. "I'd like to try them out." If he had still been editing his magazine, I'm sure there would have been an issue featuring a guide to handicap-friendly travel.

In Cambria, a charming seaside village midway between Los Angeles and San Francisco, Geoff waited in the car while I unloaded our luggage and the transport chair. I gulped and took a deep breath when I saw the handicap sign on the hotel-room door for the first time, knowing we'd reached another turning point. I thought of the handicap signs posted in parking lots, restrooms and buses that were for "other people" and felt a chill that they were now meant for us. But once inside, I checked out the roll-in shower and felt nothing but relief. There was space for the wheelchair next to the toilet and grip bars on the walls. Convenience and safety features, including risers on the toilet and chairs, enhanced our stay immeasurably.

For some fifteen years, we had a sacred tradition: a week-long Thanksgiving road trip up Highway One along California's glorious coastline to

Mendocino. While we varied the itinerary somewhat each year, we always arranged to stop at "Grandpa Deetjen's" rustic inn (Deetjen's Big Sur Inn)—where *I Jesu Navn*, the Norwegian table prayer, hangs on the dining room wall—and requested our favorite cabin deep in the woods, which came with its own resident cat.

Another custom, no matter the weather conditions, was a picnic lunch the day before Thanksgiving on a rocky bluff above the Pacific Ocean. We'd spend the day hiking in the hills, carrying backpacks stocked with champagne, sausage, bread, fruit, cheese and chocolate. A rushing creek wound through the rocky terrain, cascading over boulders and flowing into an icy stream close to our trail. We'd wedge the bottle of champagne among the rocks to settle and cool while we set out our lunch, then sit on the bluff eating while watching birds swoop over the ocean. Geoff would toss some breadcrumbs, and inevitably a seagull arrived—*his* seagull, he always insisted, jesting that the same one found us every year.

A sunny day was a bonus, but we never let rain and wind stop us. On our trip in 2008, we took the chilly drizzle in stride, although we curtailed our usual long hike; Geoff could no longer manage it in any event. Instead, we donned boots and waterproof jackets to trek a short distance along a woodsy path that led to a panoramic view of surging ocean and pounding surf. Settling under a heavy canopy of pine boughs to keep dry, we opened a split of champagne and lunched on cheese, salami, bread and fruit.

Soon another guest joined us, a plump seagull that looked awfully familiar to Geoff. Edging closer, the bird cocked his head, sizing up his chance of cadging his own lunch. We watched him strutting around, nabbing breadcrumbs before swooping off. "Hey there, fella. See you next year!" Geoff laughed.

I hoped that would be the case but wondered how many more Thanksgiving trips up the coast we would have together. Another thought came close behind: *However many, we'll make the most of each one.*

Chapter Six

Following the advice of our neurologist, I looked for ways to keep Geoff physically and mentally active. I assisted him in writing an article for our homeowner's association newsletter about film star Jacqueline Bisset, who lived in our neighborhood. We both knew her somewhat, since she and I had once played sisters in a motion picture and she'd posed for a *Los Angeles* magazine cover. I joined the interview as Geoff's notetaker, and afterward, he dictated the article to me. It made for a delightful lead story in the newsletter.

Geoff was so enlivened by the accomplishment that I enthusiastically signed us up for the Plato Society, a peer-learning program at UCLA that coordinated independent study groups on a wide variety of subjects. We chose Women of the Left Bank as our topic for the first semester, meeting on Tuesday mornings to discuss literary figures from 1920s Paris—which afforded us another excuse to travel, this time back to an era and place we both loved. Over the course of fourteen weeks, Geoff would make a presentation on Janet Flanner and I would lead a discussion on Djuna Barnes, which meant tackling lengthy reading lists throughout the course to prepare for in-depth three-hour sessions.

Ideally, Geoff and I would have joined separate study groups, but with his mobility issues, I had to be on hand to assist him. The rigorous intellectual demands of the Plato Society attracted retired academics, doctors, attorneys and other accomplished professionals, many considerably older than us, who relished stimulating, competitive discussion. With his literary background and ready wit, Geoff would have been in his element in this scholarly forum, but his increasing speech difficulties put him at considerable disadvantage. It was hard for him to take a back seat when he'd once been so deft at debate. He also struggled with reading and writing, but fortunately was already well acquainted with Janet Flanner's work. I helped him prepare his notes, and we spent days rehearsing his presentation, which was very well received.

On the heels of our Plato experience, we entered a "new normal" that I didn't recognize at first was Geoff's emotional response to his increasing physical limitations. I tried to include him in the few outside activities I continued to do, including volunteering at the homeless program at my church, where I served lunch on Monday afternoons. I brought him with me on two occasions, but I didn't foresee that assisting in any manner required coordination he no longer had. He sat on the sidelines acting as a greeter, a demoralizing reminder of his frustrating experience at the HIV/AIDS food-distribution warehouse. In attempting to keep him active and socially engaged, I'd managed to make him feel even more marginalized and useless.

Coupled with that was the inevitable fact that Geoff had no social outlets that didn't include me. I was the facilitator, always on hand, always assisting and trying to do so as unobtrusively as possible to make our lives appear normal when that wasn't the case. When we were among friends, I'd sometimes anticipate when Geoff was having difficulty saying something and jump in to say it for him, as though I were his translator. Or I would attempt to steer conversation to him so he could respond with a story—which left him feeling patronized. Plainly put, I could do no right.

Geoff was overwhelmed by the rapid deterioration in his physical condition, but he wouldn't talk with me about his feelings. I couldn't blame him for being resentful and irritable at times, but it still hurt when he took it out on me. I reminded myself that my mother, too, had tested and bullied, blaming her frustration on the person most handy. Similarly with Geoff, I knew the ravages of the disease, the medications and his feelings of anxiety and futility all played roles in his bouts of ill-temper, but I was at a loss to deal with it. No amount of reassurance or gentle humor would pull him out of a sulk. If he didn't sleep well and was tired during the day, it only added to his irritability.

One day, when we were both on edge and he'd been particularly sulky, I made his favorite soup, Manhattan clam chowder, for lunch. I'd barely set the bowl on the table when he shoved it onto the floor. I reacted angrily, but saw in his hurt look that his action was accidental, that he'd only been reaching for a spoon and couldn't control the movement of his hand.

Geoff had recently begun a new round of medications—most of them meant to treat conditions he didn't actually have, on the theory that he might benefit from their effects on aspects of his disease. He would occasionally become alarmed when seeing a television commercial for one these drugs. One particular medication he took was generally prescribed to patients with memory and cognitive disorders. "So now I'm losing my marbles, too!" he fumed.

One of the medications helped him stop slurring words. But in its place, he developed a peculiar pattern of speech in which he would rapidly repeat a phrase three times, such as "stop, stop, stop" or "can't talk, can't talk, can't talk."

In the car on the way to the grocery store, Geoff suddenly became agitated and shouted, "Take me home, take me home, take me home."

Startled, I reached for his hand to calm him, but he didn't want to be touched. I pulled into a parking space and waited quietly until his agitation passed. I had no idea what caused his outburst, but it was frightening to imagine Geoff becoming so distressed that he'd try opening the car door while I was driving—or demand to be let off an airplane while we were in flight.

At home one evening Geoff slammed his fist on the table and said, "You hate me, you hate me, you hate me."

I calmly covered his hand with mine and said, "I love you, I love you, I love you," then burst into tears when he pulled away. Within minutes, his sullenness vanished, and we sat together watching television as though nothing untoward had occurred. As raw as my nerves were dealing with his moodiness, what Geoff was going through was worse: he was experiencing terrifying physical changes that seemed incomprehensible. He had no idea what to expect next, nor did I.

As always, the antidote was travel.

Life is perfect, I wrote in my journal on Thanksgiving of 2009. We set out on our five-day trip up the coast in beautiful weather: crystal-clear skies, sunny and warm. We stayed overnight near the Hearst Castle at the Cavalier Oceanfront Resort, where the handicap rooms are state-of-the-art, safe and beautifully designed. In the late afternoon, we took a short walk to picnic at a favorite spot with a view of the ocean. We lingered, watching the sunset, and returned to our room just as twilight descended.

In the evening, we sat in armchairs near the fireplace, talking and listening to music. The following morning, I was able to bathe and dress Geoff, give him his medications and let him relax in a comfortable chair looking out on the ocean while I took my time getting myself ready. The restaurant adjoining the inn has Geoff's favorite buckwheat pancakes and apple-smoked bacon. By 9:30 a.m. we were on the road, and we arrived in Big Sur a couple hours later.

Our Thanksgiving road trip up the California coast was, as always, a mix of the familiar with new stops Geoff wanted to explore. But we were also discovering ways to better cope with his increasing physical limitations, just as he had done years earlier with Barbara on these trips. Frequent stops were essential to keep him from stiffening up, but they also meant that we visited the roadside observation points and places of historical significance that we'd whizzed past on previous trips. This time the Indian summer weather was gorgeous, a great improvement over the bleak clouds and cold mist that dampened our previous year's picnic.

Geoff napped while I explored the woodsy bluff, finding the ideal sunlit spot overlooking a rocky cove and a stunning expanse of shimmering ocean. When he awoke, we walked the short distance to the mound of smooth boulders, where Geoff could sit comfortably and look out on the ocean while we ate. By the time we'd enjoyed our leisurely picnic and returned to our cabin, he was exhausted. He napped again while I set out on a hike along the cliffs.

Geoff was awake and ready for Happy Hour when I returned. At his suggestion, I packed the cruise brochures with the split of champagne in my backpack, and we strolled up the short path to a lichen-covered bench under a canopy of spruce branches. The sun glimmered on the distant horizon as we sat sipping champagne and looking out on the ocean swelling into the cove.

I opened a brochure on Geoff's lap and paged through, feeling considerable relief that if we were to sign up for the South American cruise we were considering, I would at least be familiar with the ship. We'd sailed aboard the same ship to the Greek Isles and a sister ship on our Baltic cruise. I knew the stateroom configuration would accommodate Geoff's handicap needs, and I knew I could rely on the ship's medical staff because they'd given him excellent care on prior trips. Yet I was still reluctant to book the twenty-one-day cruise, longer than any of our others. What if, in the two months before departure, he became too immobile for me to care for on my own? I was also concerned that, far from home, we could face a "new normal" in his physical or mental condition that I wouldn't be able to handle.

As we sipped champagne and watched the brilliant sunset, Geoff started humming "Girl From Ipanema." I laughed and told him, "You should be so lucky!"

It was clear Geoff already saw himself cruising from Valparaíso, Chile, to Rio de Janeiro, Brazil, and I was more than aware of the January deadline when I had to confirm our tentative reservations. I glanced at Geoff, his face reflecting the splash of copper and magenta blazing on the horizon, and knew I couldn't disappoint him. Even as the air cooled and the gloaming was upon us, neither of us wanted to go inside, both of us lulled by the sounds of lapping waves and chirping crickets.

As daylight grew duskier, I hurried inside to get Geoff's jacket, concerned he was feeling the chill. I returned less than a minute later but found him trembling in terror, afraid I had abandoned him in the dark. His eyes were anxious, his face pale. While I tried to reassure him, I had trouble reassuring myself out of the fear that an episode like this would happen when we were far from home, traveling among strangers.

On December 31, 2009, I wrote in my journal: I slipped and almost fell while shampooing Geoff's hair and vented my frustration in a torrent of cursing that made him laugh.

"I know," he said. "And it will get worse." I felt so bad. What if I'd taken him down with me! Afterward, I sat on the couch with him and read a chapter aloud from *Pops*, the terrific biography of Louis Armstrong by Terry Teachout that I gave Geoff for Christmas. We spent most of the afternoon sitting together. I'm grateful for this time we have. It's been a year of change, and I'm fearful of what's ahead. But we'll handle it together and hope for the best.

We're going to South America . . . "If not now, when?"

Once Geoff's neurologist assured me that our trip wouldn't make us miss out on recruitment for either of two potential clinical drug trials, both in their last stages of gaining approval, I confirmed our South American cruise for mid-January 2010 and acquired visas for Brazil.

Geoff was entirely wrapped up in anticipating the cruise. Perhaps with images of the young and lovely girl from Ipanema sashaying in his head, he told me not to worry about him in South America. He'd do fine on his own, and I should just go off and enjoy myself.

This was not a practical option and far from anything I could imagine taking place. In view of Geoff's physical limitations, I needed to plan for every contingency. Weather alone was a huge consideration. In various ports along our route, we would have to factor in temperatures ranging from the mid-forties to ninety-plus degrees Fahrenheit and prepare for rain, both icy and tropical. With those variables in mind, we decided not to reserve a tour package. Instead, we could remain flexible, choosing suitable port excursions daily depending on weather and how Geoff was feeling.

For weeks I searched medical supply stores and the Internet for equipment for the cruise. Geoff was capable of walking with my help, but for shore exploration he would need a wheelchair. I discovered a collapsible transport chair that weighed only twelve pounds and could be taken aboard the aircraft. I ordered one in flaming fire-engine red.

Because I would be handling all the luggage by myself, I was determined to travel with only two large checked bags. I limited myself to one carry-on shoulder bag between us because I knew I'd have my hands full taking care of Geoff and the transport chair. I measured carefully and discovered I could fit a plastic commode/bath chair, with secure but removable screw-in legs, into one of the two large pieces of checked luggage. Once I packed all the other necessary medical supplies in the spaces around the collapsible bath chair, I had little room left for our clothing and my own personal needs. However, I knew there would be laundry facilities aboard ship. Besides, since I would be in charge of all our gear, I was better off taking as little as possible with us.

It was serendipitous that I had a chance to road test our travel and handicap gear prior to the South America excursion. A team of Canadian filmmakers were working on a documentary based on an investigative piece I'd written for *Opera News* magazine about Swedish soprano Birgit Nilsson, who was stalked by a fan for nearly a decade. *The Star and the Stalker* (in production) was scheduled to shoot for three days in San Francisco, where I would do on-camera interviews and stand-up pieces in various locations that included the War Memorial Opera House and several private homes. Misty rain and chill temperatures reminded me that south of the equator we would need rain gear and warm sweaters. But I was thrilled that the collapsible bath chair, transport chair and various travel-size grooming items were all serviceable in the constricted space in the motel room.

I recalled Geoff's stories about traveling with Barbara, who was confined to a wheelchair during her latter years with MS. He told me people always seemed surprised that they looked so happy and seemed to have so much fun together, and that, in turn, made everyone want to be around them. He claimed that if you didn't think of a disability as burdensome and didn't let it get in the way of enjoyment, people responded with a willingness to accommodate you. He also noted that Barbara, an attractive, elegant woman, was attentive to her grooming because she figured if you looked nice, people treated you better—and she was probably on to something.

Geoff joked about not wanting to look like "an old geezer with a stained shirt," and I made sure he always looked his best. He remained in a better mood if his bathing and dressing routines were handled smoothly and efficiently, so I essentially rehearsed for a full week before our departure. I packed a grooming bag with only what was required and chose clothing I could easily help him get on and off. My great coup was finding a J. Peterman jacket, warm and waterproof, that had an abundance of pockets and resembled a safari jacket. But I also packed his good English blazer and a pair of dress pants for the special evenings aboard ship, knowing how much it enforced Geoff's self-image to be well-dressed and well-groomed.

I proceeded to pack and repack our single carry-on, cramming it with medications and whatever provisions we might need in the event of flight delays or lost luggage. My foresight was rewarded when a combination of bad weather and equipment malfunction delayed our flight to Chile. We hadn't even left Los Angeles before I was relying on my emergency supplies of medications, disposable underwear, antacids, wipes, and chocolates. Keeping Geoff safe, comfortable and in a good mood throughout our long flight to South America was no easy matter, but we even managed a trip to the bathroom in the middle of the night without incident. Geoff was so amused by my contortions inside the tiny lavatory that we were both laughing as we returned to our seats.

Despite traveling some six thousand miles and making it through an extended flight of more than twelve hours, we were both in high spirits when we reached our ship. The transport chair had done its job providing a safe seat for Geoff while I handled customs, immigration, baggage and our ground transit. I was enormously relieved when we made it on board without mishap or injury and our cabin was just as I had envisioned it. While he rested, I unpacked, grateful nothing on my checklist had been left behind. The transport chair folded into a corner of the closet, handy for use in onshore excursions, and the bath chair fit in the shower stall but could be easily disassembled and stored when not in use. I was determined that our cabin not take on the appearance of an invalid's care room, distracting us from a carefree holiday.

When he awoke from his nap, Geoff squeezed my hand and confided he'd been concerned about being up to the trip. Now that he was safely on board, he was brimming with excitement and eager to stroll the upper deck as our ship left the dock. His happy grin made me wonder if I should keep him on a continuous cruise.

Geoff's good spirits carried through our first day on open water, despite rough seas that kept many seasick passengers confined to their cabins. As the ship rocked and rolled, Geoff was amused to see that people able to venture out were gripping the railings and struggling as much as he to stay on their feet. Even though we were both well, I took no chances and requested crewmembers to assist when necessary. Otherwise, with dining rooms and decks virtually to ourselves, we explored the ship with me wheeling Geoff in his transport chair.

The Horizon Room, furnished with cozy armchairs, afforded us a panoramic view of the fjords as we cruised the southern reaches of Chile. Enjoying coffee or cocktails, we'd gaze at the wondrous snow-capped mountains illuminated by the midnight sun as our ship sailed through fog-shrouded waters.

I was disappointed that our first port, Puerto Montt, could only be reached by tender and that all of the shore excursions were unsuitable for Geoff. However, we'd been together constantly for days, and Geoff, content to have time to himself, suggested I go ashore on my own. He was more than happy to sit propped up by pillows, remote control in hand, watching cable news in our cabin. I was a bit uneasy leaving him alone, but our steward promised to look in on him while I was gone.

By midmorning I reached the quay and strolled into the village marketplace, enjoying the warm, sunny weather and the open stalls displaying produce, fish and meat, eggs and cheeses, flowers and all sorts of homemade foods new to me. But by the time I reached the fishing boats at the far end of the quay, I felt such an urgency to return to the ship that I almost ran back to the dock.

Geoff appeared to be napping, but as soon as he heard me enter the room, he looked up, his eyes fearful. My breath caught in alarm when I saw his bloodied pillow, but he quickly assured me that he was all right, he hadn't fallen.

I gently lifted his head onto my lap and saw bloody scratches on his cheek, his brow scraped raw. His body was warm and feverish, yet he was shaking as though chilled. I apologized over and over for having left him alone, but he insisted I wasn't to blame. After cleaning his face with a damp cloth, I applied antiseptic cream and assessed the damage. His scratches were superficial, but patches of raw skin looked as though they'd blister.

He explained that he'd wanted to adjust his eyeglasses, but his hand started to involuntarily scratch his face, and he couldn't stop. "My hand does what it wants to," he told me. It wasn't until he'd managed to shove his glasses under the pillow that he was able to regain control. I found his eyeglasses there, slightly bent and the lenses bloody. I was glad I'd packed spare glasses, but felt miserable that I'd let this happen. Geoff saw my reaction and said, "Not your fault. Not your fault. Not your fault."

I later reflected that we'd experienced a moment of rare insight on Geoff's part: he was both aware of his behavior and capable of describing what occurred. Often he was oblivious to these involuntary actions, looking at me bewildered, unable to comprehend what had happened to him. But I regretted not recognizing that he needed eye drops. His eyes were sore and dry because he was losing control of blinking, causing him to rub and scratch his lids. I felt very much responsible for the pain he'd suffered while I'd strolled through a marketplace.

I sensed Geoff's anguish, too, surely recalling his own years as a caregiver and knowing how necessary it was for each of us to have time alone. We sat on the edge of the bed, both of us feeling miserable, until Geoff said, "I'm hungry. Lunch?"

He gave me one of his manic Jack Nicholson grins and added, "I'm going to have a beer, too."

On the cruise, I watched for signs of behavioral changes, some of which, like involuntary finger tapping or excessive yawning, were of little consequence. More troubling was Geoff's nonstop squirming, which began on the third day of our voyage and became increasingly disruptive. He was unable to sit still, his restlessness becoming so severe that he would slide out of a chair or tip it over. He constantly asked to be "reseated," but no matter how many times I adjusted him, he was still uncomfortable. Our antics trying to reposition him were almost comical, but as his agitation escalated I grew desperate, afraid that he would injure himself. Then, as frequently happened with these quirky episodes, the restlessness suddenly stopped.

As often accompanied the onset of new physical changes, Geoff's mood swings were unpredictable. Aboard ship I remained hyperalert to his emotional state to avoid a public scene that could spoil the enjoyment of other passengers or cause embarrassment to us. Although crewmembers and fellow passengers were quick to offer help by holding a door or stepping aside in a narrow corridor, we didn't want to appear needy. We preferred not to be seated at group tables because Geoff was generally unable to join in conversation and required my assistance eating. Rather than cause distraction, we arranged to sit by ourselves at quiet corner tables where I could cut up his food and help him eat. I never rushed, finding pleasure in this quiet, private time together.

By the fifth day of our voyage, Geoff was thriving on bracing sea air, exercise, wonderful meals and the ever-changing scenery. His face was fully healed, his mood swings were tempered and his gait improved so much we rarely used the transport chair. I was certain my constant companionship and full attention to his needs contributed to avoiding the medical conditions I'd most dreaded, including diarrhea and constipation, adverse reactions to medication, choking and falling—but the strain of staying alert was intense. When I started feeling too overwhelmed, I would find a safe place to leave Geoff on his own so I could have a few minutes to myself. Often a brisk walk on the deck was enough, but sometimes I needed solitude to shed a few tears—which wasn't easy aboard a cruise ship with scant privacy.

Occasionally I would leave Geoff in the company of a man who had struck up a conversation with him in the Horizon Room. The two would chat over afternoon coffee, which gave me a chance to go off on my own. I sensed that while this passenger clearly enjoyed getting together with Geoff, he also did so as a means of giving me some free time.

If the weather was good and the port accessible without a tender, we'd disembark and explore, made much easier thanks to the transport chair. Usually we'd make our way to the end of the quay and hire a private driver for a tour. If the driver spoke English and the transport chair could be folded into the trunk, I'd negotiate a rate, and off we'd go for the day.

At Geoff's urging, I booked myself on a catamaran excursion to Laguna San Rafael to see the glaciers on my birthday. The trip across rough, frigid waters would not have been suitable for Geoff, and we prearranged for his shipboard friend to join him in the Horizon Room after lunch. By midafternoon, I was on the catamaran chugging toward the San Valentín glacier, knowing Geoff was in safe hands. I'd been told rain drenched the area thirteen out of fourteen days, but I struck it lucky with brilliant sunny skies. The imposing blue-glass icebergs were stunning from a distance and spectacular a stone's throw from the boat. I couldn't have dreamed of a more adventurous, thrilling birthday treat.

I was alarmed when I didn't find Geoff in the Horizon Room when I returned, but a steward told me he'd requested assistance returning to our stateroom. I felt a surge of relief when I found him propped in bed watching Turner Classic Movies and looking very pleased with himself for managing so well in my absence. He was in great spirits as I helped him dress for dinner, clearly determined to give me a special day in the only way he still could. Knowing that touched me deeply. My husband had little means of demonstrating his affection, unable any longer to romance me with flowers and sweet gifts. The love in his eyes conveyed his tender feelings and let me know he was still there for me.

That evening we dined in the stylish Tuscany Room at a corner table the waiters obligingly rearranged so I sat looking out on the lagoon and could unobtrusively assist Geoff with eating. Thick forest framed glimmering fjords and majestic snowcapped mountains glistening in the pearly glow of the midnight sun. We indulged in a fine red wine with a delicious dinner, capped with chocolate cake and a modest number of lit candles. We toasted nature's glorious scenery and a day made memorable by Geoff's wish to make it special.

But stormy clouds heavy with pelting rain darkened our room the following morning as the ship juddered in the swelling waves. Gloom seemed to settle over us, too. Geoff hadn't slept well and seemed listless and morose. His breathing was ragged, and he had difficulty finding his balance, so I kept him in bed propped up with pillows. Perhaps he'd partied too much the night before, even a few sips of wine too much for him. I curled up next to him, reading until he fell asleep, the warmth of his body next to mine a tender comfort.

Quiet times such as these filled me with aching sadness, knowing I was losing him and unable to imagine a future without him. As frail as he was, we could still share new experiences and enjoy our companionship. How could I live in a world without him?

We sailed into Ushuaia, the southernmost port on our itinerary, on a crisp, clear morning perfect for a day of sightseeing. After most passengers had disembarked, I enlisted crewmembers to assist Geoff down the ramp in his transport chair, and we set off on our own. When we reached the quay, I surveyed the steep inclines and narrow, twisting sidewalks in town and knew that, unless we could hire a car and driver for a private tour, we would be spending our day confined to the pier. Craig and Barbara, a couple we'd spent some time with aboard ship, strolled up to us with the same thought in mind. Together we found an obliging driver who spoke English and had a car roomy enough for the four of us.

The driver, garrulous and accommodating, took us to remote beaches and breathtaking roadside vantage points in Tierra del Fuego National Park that couldn't accommodate tour buses. The terrain was too rugged for the transport chair, but Geoff was able to walk with my support along a mossy forest path to a swampy stretch of wooded area with a beaver dam. Later, we traversed a narrow, rickety bridge to a strip of land where we could look toward Antarctica, directly across the Drake Passage!

That afternoon, back in port, our driver dropped us at a restaurant where we ate king crab and shared a bottle of local wine with our friends before returning to the ship.

Emboldened by the successful outing, when the cruise ship reached our port in the Falkland Islands the following morning, Geoff was game to board the tender for the choppy ride ashore. This time we were on our own with no one to assist us with the steep ramp to the pier. The small wheels on the transport chair weren't designed to handle the hilly terrain, but the air was invigorating, the smell of the sea intoxicating. We traversed the oceanfront promenade from Christ Church Cathedral, Thatcher Drive and the war memorial to the Government House and back, managing to avoid acquiring penguin souvenirs along the way. Before returning to the ship, I indulged Geoff by pushing him up a steep slope to the Globe Tavern where he could enjoy a few sips of Guinness.

Geoff had been in good humor throughout the day, getting a kick out of watching patrons play darts in the pub and teasing me when I swore each time the transport wheels got stuck in cracked pavement. I reveled in times like these when whatever struggle we faced traveling was worth it—if anything, the additional effort gave us a greater sense of accomplishment. Instead of longing for the days when Geoff would have been walking alongside me or playing darts himself, we found pleasure in what we still could do. As we headed back to the pier, Geoff playfully called out, "Mush," to urge me to push faster so we wouldn't miss the tender. The two of us laughed when the wheels jammed again, his high spirits a joyful reminder of the fun we had together, making me glad we'd taken the trip.

Back aboard ship, we sat wrapped in blankets on deck chairs, enjoying the tangy ocean air. I read and Geoff napped as we sailed out of port into open seas, the ship rocking in the swelling waves. But when he awoke, he was sulky and asked to return to our cabin. A steward helped me get him on his feet. Geoff was hungry, and I thought stopping in his favorite Terrace Café might lighten his mood. If only I'd taken him directly to the cabin and ordered room service instead.

Unfortunately, I misread signals that he'd become disoriented with the pitch and roll of the ship in open water, and my change in direction only confused him more. He reacted in panic when the elevator doors opened on a crowd of passengers, who shifted to make room for us. I wanted to wait for a less packed elevator, but the steward was already helping Geoff aboard. Squeezed into tight quarters, he became further agitated when he was unable to grasp a handrail to steady himself. The jostling, exuberant passengers were more than he could tolerate, particularly when one of them loudly exclaimed about the glorious weather.

Snarling and waving his hands, Geoff repeated, "Glorious! Glorious! Glorious!"

I tried to soothe him, but he kept shouting, alarming the other passengers. When the doors opened on the next floor, I helped him out of the elevator, but he stumbled, lost his footing and fell against a wall, still shouting. A nearby passenger offered assistance. He took Geoff's arm and helped me get him back to the safety of our room, where he sank into a chair, ashen and trembling.

I closed the door and broke down sobbing, warning Geoff we'd be kicked off the ship if he behaved badly toward other passengers, who were only being kind and friendly. He responded with more repetitious outbursts, shouting, "Sorry. Sorry. Sorry. Can't help it. Can't help it. Can't help it."

"Then don't do it, do it, do it, damn it!"

I regretted my response as soon as the words fell from my mouth. I knew he couldn't help himself, that erratic behavior was part of his disease. Rapid mood shifts, angry outbursts and the repetition of words and phrases were endemic to the condition. I was ashamed for having overreacted—but I couldn't help it, either!

I pulled myself together and put a consoling hand on my husband's shoulder, asking him if he was still hungry.

"No. I want to go home," he said, a scowl on his face.

I burst into laughter, telling him we were stuck on board unless he felt like swimming.

Geoff managed a crooked smile. In that case, he said, he was still hungry.

For the rest of the evening, we snuggled on the couch watching a screwball comedy on Turner Classic Movies and eating salads and poached salmon from room service. Though the tension had dissipated, I still felt jumpy, chiding myself for not picking up on the first signs of a mood change. But Geoff's outburst had also tested the limits of my tolerance for public disgrace. While he slept soundly, I brooded, dredging up hurts, slights and long-unresolved misunderstandings from the whole of our marriage.

But when Geoff awoke, his leg curled against mine, I saw in his troubled gaze that he recalled the events of the evening before. I responded to his whispered apology with reassurances and we lingered in an embrace. Instead of the rage that had robbed me of sleep, I felt gratitude for the time we still had together and sorrow that we'd never again be the way we were.

One afternoon not long after, a man standing next to me at a dessert buffet startled me by asking if I was accompanying my father on the trip. I was astonished that Geoff, only a few years older than me, could possibly be mistaken for my father. I glanced over at our table, where he sat with hunched shoulders, his face slack—and I saw him as others did. In my mind, he was still the handsome, vibrant man I'd married, and he always would be.

I told the man that my husband had a neurological disease that affected his mobility. He nodded toward his wife seated nearby, a trim, attractive woman I'd often seen walking around the upper deck, and told me she'd had cancer for five years and was taking chemo even while on the cruise. "Every day we have together is a gift."

Chapter Seven

In the months following the trip to South America, Geoff's physical condition deteriorated so rapidly that I understood how narrowly we'd almost missed being able to take the cruise. He was soon unable to walk or feed himself and required so much assistance that I couldn't leave him alone at all. Candelaria, our longtime housekeeper, looked after Geoff every Wednesday while I raced out for grocery shopping and other vital errands. Otherwise, the two of us were together around the clock, rarely venturing out or getting together with friends.

Geoff missed having quiet suppers with a friend or two in the garden or kitchen. To alleviate our growing isolation, I introduced late-afternoon Happy Hour, a time when our family and friends could drop by for coffee or drinks. The master bedroom became our cocktail lounge with the addition of a small round table and chairs and the removal of any sign of medical equipment. Geoff's voice had grown very faint, so I bought an inexpensive voice amplifier with a headset and sponge-covered mic that he dubbed Madonna. How wonderful to hear his voice again! He delighted in doing sound checks before guests arrived and could once again join in conversation.

Even as Geoff grew frailer, the socializing lifted his spirits—and, to my surprise, his appetite for travel was undiminished. I knew that South America had been our last major trip, but I indulged his blissful denial by tentatively booking a Caribbean cruise while dealing with the alternate reality of home hospice care. Geoff clearly fit the criteria and I applied for it, assured that the palliative care would not affect his enrollment in a phase II drug trial.

Thanksgiving of 2010 marked the beginning of hospice care, and with it came a deluge of paperwork, equipment, medication and rotating staff, including a visit by a nurse once a week, a health aide twice a week to assist with bathing, and a doctor on call. The reality of all that it involved, including having oxygen equipment and restricted drugs on hand, unsettled me. Despite reassurances from Geoff's doctors, I worried that it was too soon for hospice. Was I doing the right thing for his safety and comfort or hastening the end?

My fear was unfounded: the palliative care Geoff received was so beneficial that his general health improved. He felt more secure with a trained aide helping bathe and dress him, and he benefited from more closely monitored medications and breathing treatments. He'd rebounded significantly enough that he wanted more than anything to be in New York over the Christmas holidays—and I wanted to make it happen. The hospice team left the decision to us, assuring me we could reinstate care after the start of the new year. I booked our flight using miles and upgrades, well aware that friends and family thought I was completely out of my mind.

Our flight to New York on December 16 went remarkably smoothly, with Geoff in good spirits throughout the trip. My carry-on was packed with treats in case he got restless, but Geoff seemed content to recline in his seat, snug under a blanket, looking out the window. We both felt festive, a feeling that only increased when we arrived at our apartment to find family members there to greet us, including my brother Orlyn, who'd arrived from Minneapolis hours earlier, and my nephew Tom and his wife, Barbara, visiting from Rhode Island. They'd decorated a tree, bought flowers and had wine and cheese waiting for us. Orlyn and Tom had also assembled a new wheelchair that I'd ordered online, and they had it ready to use when we all went for dinner in the neighborhood. The following day, my nephew wheeled Geoff to see the Rockefeller Center Christmas tree before we all met for dinner and an evening of jazz at Birdland. Though none of us mentioned it, we knew this would likely be our last Christmas, if not our final visit to New York together. My family could not have given us a more joy-filled gift.

As much as I got used to each "new normal," it seemed impossible to anticipate what the next significant change would be. The home care aide I had arranged for New York failed to show up, and the agency could not supply a replacement over the holidays. I struggled on my own to give Geoff the care that our hospice team had provided, and hadn't predicted the effect jet lag, travel fatigue and the shift in the weather would have. He was too weak to walk even a few steps, and I had difficulty transferring him to a chair, where he could sit up only when propped with pillows. At night, he started hallucinating, thrashing and speaking nonsensically. A recurring delusion was his fear of missing a flight to Moscow; another that he had to stop someone stealing cartoons, insisting that "justice must be done!"

Often I couldn't understand his manic, garbled rants. Cupping his face in my hands, I tried to soothe his panic, assuring him we were safe, with no plans to go anywhere. But at times he became so agitated that it was difficult to keep him from shifting himself off the bed. Unable to turn over or adjust his body, he couldn't sleep and became even more disoriented. On one occasion, I awoke just after midnight to see that he had a foot on the floor, was seated almost upright and was on the verge of falling over. He insisted it was time to get up, but I opened the curtains to show him it was still dark outside.

As I lay wide awake next to him, trembling with nerves and exhaustion, I pleaded with him to let me sleep at night so I could care for him during the day—though I knew he couldn't help hallucinating, and scolding him for it made no sense.

"I'll soon be gone," he said. "Then I won't bother you."

The remark caught me off guard, cutting deeply. However frustrated or fatigued I felt, I couldn't let myself take it out on him. But it struck me this was the first time he'd made reference to dying, to leaving me. I assured him I wanted him with me forever, and curled closer, hugging his body to mine, not ever wanting to let go.

The night terrors convinced me that Geoff ought to be back in Los Angeles—but how could I get him there? The thought of taking a flight with Geoff in his present condition, prone to outbursts and hallucinations, was terrifying. I even had the rash notion of renting a car and tearing across the country despite dire blizzard warnings.

Before I could make any such foolish decisions, Geoff rebounded again. One morning, after several unbearable sleepless nights, he woke up smiling and fully coherent, asking for pancakes. Later that day we had lunch in a neighborhood restaurant and talked about our plans for the holidays. On Christmas Eve, we joined carolers singing at Irving Berlin's former house in Beekman Place. Bundled up against the chill of the night, I wrapped my arms around Geoff, held him close and sang "White Christmas" under a star-filled sky.

Aside from those rocky first nights, our holiday was a magical blend of everything we savored about Christmas in New York, including snowy days spent at home in our apartment. After friends, who had joined us for a New Year's Eve dinner, left and Geoff was safely tucked in bed, I took a short walk to the end of our street. Geoff's remark that he'd soon be gone had lingered in my mind for days. It was uncharacteristic of him, and I wondered if he even remembered saying it. I instinctively knew not to bring it up, but hoped if he mentioned it again I could encourage him to open up about his feelings.

Looking across the East River, where the Pepsi-Cola sign sparkled like a giant Christmas bauble, my eyes watered as I made a promise to myself to be patient and kind and treasure the precious moments we had left together. *No harsh words you'll regret, because you can't take them back, not ever.*

Chapter Eight

One morning in late January, not quite a month after our return from New York, Geoff awoke seemingly revitalized, and I imagined that the drug he'd been taking in the phase II clinical trial was a magic potion that had done its job. His appetite was robust. Once again I was able to walk him from the bed to the recliner. His voice was vibrant, even without using his Madonna. There were no signs of confusion or weakness. He seemed in a hurry, showing impatience if I couldn't retrieve books and papers he wanted quickly enough.

I took advantage of his newfound strength to ask if he'd like my help in organizing his *Los Angeles* magazine archives, which he planned to donate to the UCLA library. He said the file drawers were locked, and he'd forgotten where the key was. He told me not to bother looking for it because I'd never find it.

He seemed so vigorous that I felt comfortable leaving him in Candelaria's care while I attended my birthday lunch with book club friends at a nearby restaurant. When I arrived back home some ninety minutes later, I was astonished at all Geoff had accomplished in my absence—and dismayed. He'd inveigled our housekeeper to help him clear out file drawers in his office. Bulging black plastic bags and cartons stuffed with papers and the contents of desk drawers were piled at the bottom of the stairs. Geoff was settled back in his recliner, legs crossed, his eyes bright and alert when I entered the bedroom.

"You must've found the key. Why didn't you wait for me to help you?"

"I remembered where I put it," he said. "I threw away some stuff. Don't bother looking in the bags."

The exchange was surreal, given that Geoff had struggled to converse for well over a year. I told him I was concerned about what he'd thrown away and would have to look through the bags, but promised I would not read or look at anything he didn't want me to see.

As soon as I opened the first bag, I started finding essential documents, including our marriage license and the original deed to the house. In another bag I came across a box with a piece of jewelry intended as a gift for me years earlier that he'd stashed away and thought was lost. An accompanying card read: *K—With all my love, G.*

He seemed surprised I'd found the bracelet but wasn't at all contrite. I was furious but tried to make light of the situation, thanking him for the timely birthday gift that had almost made it to a dumpster. I was rewarded with a grudging smile. I set aside documents and items important to keep but discarded the rest as he'd intended. He clearly resented my interference, his wrath evident in his icy silence when I served him dinner and helped him to bed that night.

Had I recognized the signs, I could have handled everything more gracefully. That night, for the first time in weeks, Geoff slept soundly through the night. I awoke in the early morning to hear him murmuring, "What's holding us up from leaving?"

"We're not going anywhere. Where do you want to go?"

"Home."

"We're home. Look out the window. That's our garden." He looked feverish, his skin clammy. "Are you all right?"

"I want to go home." He clamped his eyes shut, tears spilling onto his cheek. He began to wheeze, his breath labored. I telephoned the hospice nurse, who arrived quickly and diagnosed pneumonia. When I described his strength and vitality only the day before, she said, "It goes that way, sometimes. A burst of energy before the end."

"The end! No! We need to get him to the hospital!"

I terminated hospice care and called 911. Paramedics rushed Geoff to emergency care, where I lifted the DNR (do-not-resuscitate order) so he could be treated. Standing next to the gurney, holding his hand, I sobbed a plea not to leave me. After what had taken place the afternoon before, I was desperate for time to heal the rift between us and make amends.

I sat at his bedside throughout the long night, my eyes on Geoff, illuminated in the flickering glow of the monitors. The steady beeping was a comfort. I was mortified that I'd lashed out, demeaning him by tearing through the bags instead of trying to understand his motivation. He didn't need *things* anymore—was there any reason for me to show him that I did? All I'd managed to do was point out the irreversible divide expanding between us; he was leaving, while I was staying behind.

Upon reflection I realized that Geoff had begun a journey, this time without me. Instead of packing, he'd been discarding, leaving behind what he would not need again. I'd interrupted his mission, one that called on the last of his strength and energy to tidy up before going on his way; the impulse reminded me of my mother in her final days. The cold indifference I'd taken as a rebuke was Geoff pulling away, letting me know it was time for him to go "home."

When he awoke in the morning, there was a look of wonder in his eyes, and he appeared surprised to see me. I knew that the next time, I'd have to let him go, but I was grateful for the warmth in his smile and a chance to make amends. I wanted no regrets.

On February 9, I wrote in my journal—I've prepared Geoff the best I can for my last-minute one-day visit to Minneapolis. Aunty Pat is in hospice at North Memorial Hospital. We're so close, and I desperately want to see her before she passes. I've thought about the trip, even checked airline schedules, but Geoff is so newly out of hospital himself that I haven't wanted to make the reservations. I know if I don't make the trip now, I won't see her at all.

I wavered in my decision, the specter of regret hanging in the balance. My glamorous godmother, who trailed scents of White Shoulders perfume and Chesterfield cigarettes, had always had time for me, letting me read her racy novels and dip into her cache of exotic costume jewelry. As a schoolgirl I loved visiting the bridal shop where she worked, a fairyland of satin, lace and tulle gowns and cocktail dresses in a rainbow of colors. I never went home without fancy shopworn castoffs for games of dress up or to use as costumes in neighborhood parades, plays and pageants with playmates. How could I miss seeing my beloved Aunty Pat this one last time?

I meticulously planned my one-day trip, arranging for a friend to spend the night so that when I left for the airport at 4:45 a.m. to catch the first flight to Minneapolis, he'd be on hand for Geoff until home care aides arrived at 6:00 a.m. I'd have a scant six hours to see my aunt and visit with my sister, Sandra, who was celebrating her sixty-fifth birthday in her special-needs residence, before my return flight.

Geoff awakened just as I was leaving. I kissed him, reassured him I'd be back by evening and eased out the door, hoping he wouldn't panic at my absence. Checking in at the airport, I experienced a sense of guilt-ridden liberation to be traveling without luggage, a transport chair and the dread of getting Geoff through a TSA screening. After boarding my flight on time, I fell asleep before takeoff and didn't wake up until landing in Minneapolis. My brother Orlyn met me at the curb, and we drove directly to the hospital. Taking in the wintry vista on the way, it occurred to me that the last time I'd been in Minnesota was to accompany Geoff to the Mayo Clinic some three years earlier.

Aunty Pat, two years younger than my mother, had her own apartment in the same senior-living facility, although the two highly independent, opinionated women, who never quite got along, had lived completely separate lives. As I raced through the hospital's familiar halls to the fourth-floor palliative-care wing, I realized that Aunty Pat was in the same room my mother had been in at the end of her life. What would the sisters have made of that?

I barely recognized my aunt, her beautiful face slack and colorless. I approached her quietly, not wanting to startle her with my unexpected presence. I kissed her forehead and whispered my name, letting her know I'd come to see her. Holding her hand, I told her I loved her and that she was my fairy godmother, and I thanked her for bringing so much magic into my life. She blinked, opening her smoky-blue eyes. Crossing her fingers in a familiar gesture, she touched my cheek before drifting off again. I knew for certain I'd have no regrets and was thankful I'd made the right decision.

I arrived back home that evening to find Geoff already in bed, awake but anxious and silent. He thought I'd abandoned him even though Karen, a skilled home care aide he liked, had been with him throughout the day, reassuring him I would return. I held his hand, trying to comfort him as I told him about my visit with Aunty Pat and quick stop to see my sister on the way to the airport. I sat with him until he drifted off, feeling miserable that my day trip had been so hard on him. The following morning, he was noticeably weaker, his breathing labored, and the hospice nurse gave him nebulizer treatments to clear his lungs. I spent the day with him, rarely leaving his side, to make up for my absence the day before.

February 11—Once again I was awakened before dawn. Geoff nudged me and whispered that the car has arrived to pick us up. I could barely make out his words. I asked him how he felt.

"Bad."

"Why?"

"I'm dying."

"We all are. We just don't know when."

I stroked his cheek and gently reminded him that a close friend who was healthy when Geoff was diagnosed had since passed away. My tone was light, my whispered words meant to comfort, but I was deeply shaken.

It was the second time my husband had spoken of impending death. I shifted closer, my head on his pillow, hoping he would say more but not pressing him. With my breath warm on his cheek, my nearness provided reassurance I would always be there for him. He drifted off, and I didn't move. Gazing at the fine lines around his eyes and creases in his forehead, I imprinted them in memory, not wanting to forget the face I loved. I touched his hair, once curly and dark, now bone white and soft as duck feathers, his stubbly beard as pale as his skin. I saw him as he was now but remembered him as he once was.

I matched my breath to his, hoping to feel what he was feeling and divine his thoughts. I knew I couldn't ask him, but perhaps when he awoke again, he might share feelings about the departure he knew was coming. It was a trip he'd be taking on his own, but I wanted him to know I'd be with him until he left.

On Valentine's Day I drove to Holy Cross Cemetery to arrange burial for Geoff, the date adding even greater poignancy to a task I'd long put off. I'd been prompted to make an appointment by a hospice nurse, who had quietly suggested I organize "final arrangements." I'd been to the cemetery with Geoff when we visited his parents' graves and knew he wanted to be buried there, but didn't have a plot—which I soon learned was very pricey real estate, even with a "pre-need" discount. My humor dark, I wondered if they had closeout sales? Coupons? My mood brightened when I learned there was one plot still available in the section where his parents were buried. It seemed providential, and I signed on the dotted line, then cried all the way home.

Despite having hospice nurses rotating around the clock, I climbed into the hospital bed with Geoff at night, curling up next to him in the dark for a few hours before returning to my own bed nearby. I didn't want him to awaken in panic, alone and disoriented.

Father Gabri, the priest at my episcopal church, lifted Geoff's spirits with a Happy Hour visit late one afternoon. Raised Catholic, Father Gabri had served as an altar boy at the same Catholic church where Geoff had been an altar boy years earlier. Decades apart in age, Father Gabri reminisced with Geoff about growing up in the same Beverly Hills neighborhood. Before he left, he gave Geoff last rites.

Several close friends and family members dropped by, most sensing this could be their last visit with Geoff. He was unable to speak, and I wondered how much he comprehended, yet I understood how meaningful it was for friends and family to have those private minutes with him to say their final farewells.

On Saturday, April 2, I noted in my journal that Geoff closed his lips, refusing nourishment. He'd turned his head away after choking on even small amounts of liquid dripped in his mouth through a straw. Earlier in his illness, he'd made his wishes clear. He had expressly stated he did not want to be intubated and was adamant about not having a feeding tube. But even though he was unresponsive, I was unsettled about following through on the health directives. Was I making a mistake? Who said it's time to let him go? With his slim hold on life slipping away, I was torn.

My distress was apparent to hospice staff, who helped me understand that his body was shutting down, that prolonging the inevitable would only increase his suffering. I knew he wanted to go home. This time I couldn't interrupt his journey.

I was reminded of what Geoff told me when my mother was nearing her end: *It's her journey. Just be there for her.* He'd been there for

Barbara and knew how profound that departure was for the one staying behind as much as for the one leaving. There was no timetable; he would choose the moment.

The final farewell came on a starlit evening in mid-April. I sat at Geoff's bedside, as I had since early morning, grateful that a hospice nurse had been unable to fulfill her shift and we'd been left on our own. He'd become restless shortly after sunup, and I'd given him medication, a drop at a time under his tongue as I'd been taught. His end was near, but I knew he could still hear my voice and the birds twittering in a nest outside the window. As the medication took effect, a faint smile lifted the corner of his mouth, and his eyes flickered open, brilliant blue and lit with wonder.

His gaze was so direct, so intimate that I caught my breath, feeling a flush of shyness. He looked youthful, his skin taut and smooth, sparking memories of the man who'd won my heart decades earlier. "You're still the handsomest man I ever knew," I whispered. I held his gaze until his eyes fluttered and closed, hearing him sigh as though he, too, had been holding his breath.

I eased myself into the hospital bed, careful not to dislodge oxygen tubes. Curling my body next to his, I breathed in his musky warmth and felt the beat of my heart against his. The motorized vinyl mattress moved gently to prevent bedsores. It quivered and wheezed, a rhythmic *shush* that lulled me into a drifting reverie. I saw us as we had been in fleeting snapshots from our travels, when we'd prevail on a passerby to snap our photograph to use on Christmas cards. Geoff had pointed out how often we were photographed midway across bridges—in Paris, London, Prague, Venice, Saint Petersburg and New York's Central Park—or sitting in a pub or sidewalk café, each with a glass in hand, smiling and carefree.

We were midway on the last leg of another journey now, but would part somewhere along the way as Geoff traveled on alone. I thought about his annual springtime drives up Highway One to attend the Monterey Jazz Festival, a tradition he began during his college years. I rarely joined him on this trip, knowing how much he liked having four days by himself, immersed in music he loved. We'd walk out the door together, Geoff striding ahead wearing his customary travel garb, worn jeans and tattered safari jacket, a cap pulled low on his forehead. He'd slide behind the wheel of his convertible and begin loading the specially selected jazz CDs that would keep him company on his drive north.

Missing him already, I'd hover at the open car door making him promise to call me en route. But Geoff would only half listen as I gave him a cell phone and reminded him how to use it. After a lingering kiss, I'd wave goodbye until his car disappeared around the curve, knowing I wouldn't hear from him unless the cell phone accidentally turned on in his pocket. Then I'd hear his footsteps walking down a street, the sound of a swing band in the background. It was maddening that he couldn't hear me calling to him, but at least I knew he'd safely arrived, that he was all right. Would I somehow hear from him on this journey and know all was well?

Geoff sighed again, murmuring something I could barely hear.

"I love you, too," I whispered. I matched my breathing to his and drifted off.

Throughout that day, I remained close, playing CDs of Artie Shaw and Benny Goodman while paging through scrapbooks, the photographs illustrating my running commentary on our happy travels together. Late in the day, Geoff's breathing changed, becoming ragged and shallow. I held his hand as Artie Shaw's "Night and Day" played softly. I told him I knew this was his journey, that he wouldn't be back. I didn't want him to leave, but he couldn't let that stop him. My lips to his ear, I whispered, "I'm with you as long as you need me. Somehow, when you get there, let me know you arrived safely. I'll miss you terribly, but no tears now. You've made me strong, and I'll be fine. We'll be together again. Just save me a place at your side."

His breathing calmed, a faint whiffle fading into sudden, profound silence. I kissed Geoff's forehead, stroked his cheek and let him go where I couldn't follow. He was at peace. Tears I'd held back rolled down my cheeks, and in this moment of stillness I, too, felt at peace, thankful I'd shared this passage with him. The sharp pangs of grieving had begun with his diagnosis years earlier when I knew our life together would be cut short, but looking at the still figure of the man I loved, I was filled with gratitude that we'd had time together at all. Our romance was a gift from the moment we met to our last goodbye—and I probably wouldn't change a thing, except to ask for more time.

PART TWO

"WE COME INTO THIS WORLD ALONE AND
LEAVE IT ALONE . . ."

Chapter Nine

In those blessed moments of grace after Geoff's passing, I sat quietly, awed by the power and suddenness of death. I lingered, my hand on his brow, not wanting to move and lose that instant when life hung in a last breath. I wanted to cling to my pregrieving self when I hadn't yet lost him; to replay those last minutes when he was still with me, his flesh warm to my touch.

I sat for long minutes, the room itself chilling with night air as ice-cold grief descended on me. He was gone from my life, and I was alone. The knowledge rocked me in a tidal wave of anger and despair. *Come back! Don't leave me!* I sobbed; I made gut-wrenching sounds and felt ashamed that I wasn't keeping promises I'd only just made in Geoff's dying moments. I'd vowed to be strong, assured him I'd be fine and bid him farewell without tears. But knowing I'd never see him again—or have him hold me in his arms or feel the thump of pleasure when he walked into a room—was unbearable. That, I recognized, was the reality of grief entering my life.

A hospice nurse arrived, a remarkable young man who took charge of Geoff with compassion and tenderness. I gained strength from the nurse and began making the calls he reminded me were necessary in order to fulfill my husband's wishes. Having participated in clinical drug trials and an environmental study, Geoff had also signed on to be an organ donor, giving his brain to the Brain Bank research team at the Mayo Clinic in Jacksonville, Florida. He wanted to support CurePSP's medical research into finding a cure for prime-of-life diseases, including the progressive supranuclear palsy that had claimed his life.

Gracious friends offered to spend the night with me, but I wanted to be on my own, to sob and make all the loud, ugly sounds I'd managed to contain through one phone call after another. I listened to the heavy silence, broken only by the sound of crickets through the open window, then fell asleep.

Friends took me for Sunday lunch. Afterward, I arrived home to find florist deliveries on my doorstep. I walked in, looked at the empty lift chair we'd installed when Geoff could no longer manage stairs, and sat on the steps, blood pounding in my skull, deafening me in the terrible empty quiet. The house was so frighteningly silent.

I was startled when the doorbell rang. Assuming it was another flower delivery, I opened the door. Candelaria, who had come every Wednesday for thirty-seven years and helped Geoff care for Barbara throughout her long illness, had stopped by after church. I should have known she would come to see me. She was family, and I was grateful to find her standing there with a flower arrangement that had just been delivered. I sat back down on the stairs, crying as she made tea and offered comfort. Recently widowed herself, she understood my sobbing lament. "Come back, damn it! Just come back!"

The business of death does take a holiday; in our case it was Passover and Easter. This wasn't a time to die or get married; sanctuaries were booked to capacity with traditional holiday services. Anyone not involved in the religious end of things was on spring break. With offices closed and staff away, there was little I could accomplish. Since everything else seemed to stop, so did I.

Often I would sit idle in the garden, my hands in my lap, my thoughts free-floating. With the flush of spring in the air, the sycamore trees grew leafy, shedding the dried husks of their buds on the patio tiles. Crocuses, daffodils and freesia poked up through the earth and burst into bloom. For days I monitored the frantic goings-on in a bird's nest under the eaves, the frenzied chirping signaling new life. With the sun warm on my shoulders, the whisper of a breeze on my cheek, I felt Geoff's presence all around me as I contemplated the long summer days ahead without him.

This parcel of free time was a gift. I could be entirely on my own without demands or responsibilities. Instead of rushing to organize a funeral and memorial, I was able to reflect on fresh grief, ponder what next and cry without holding back. Throughout those days and nights, my thoughts were on Geoff and life without him. I paged through scrapbooks, each photograph transporting me to a distinct time, place and fond memory I could savor and relive.

Early one morning, I awoke to a faint rustling sound and saw that the puffy green vinyl cover on the hospital bed was quivering and gently wheezing. Perhaps the medical-transport team assigned to handle Geoff's organ donation accidentally turned the motor back on? I got up and flicked its switch off, then fell onto the hideous deflating mattress, screaming, "Come back. Just, damn it, come back!"

Then I recalled how often Geoff's cell phone would automatically turn on in his back pocket and wondered if he'd pulled off this trick to let me know all was well.

Later, a man from the hospice facility arrived to haul away all the equipment, including the hospital bed with the collapsed remains of the green mattress. While he disassembled the bed, I worked at my desk but looked up when he appeared in the doorway waving an electrical plug at me. My husband could have been electrocuted, he told me with a dark scowl. The electrical cord had been snagged in the metal lift, and with the mechanism going up and down, he could have been "crisped," as the driver put it, snapping his fingers. "Dead, just like that!"

"He is dead," I replied calmly.

"But not like that! It's not the way you want to go."

No, I agreed, it wasn't. Then it occurred to me how often I'd joined Geoff in that bed. One careless press on the remote control and we could've been crisped together. I started to laugh, telling the startled deliveryman, "Just wasn't meant to be, I guess."

"You gotta be more careful." He shook his head, coiled the electrical cord in his hands and returned to work. Geoff would've howled with laughter.

Along with wonderful memories came painful twinges of remorse. I gave in to them rather than burying them to resurface later. I came to recognize that guilt and self-recrimination play significant roles in the grieving process. I'd hoped not to have regrets, but I did, and I allowed myself to feel the full brunt of them, dwelling on a cascade of "should haves, could haves." Had I done all I could to care for Geoff, all that he would have wanted? I replayed his final days over and over, recalling our last private moments together, reminding myself it was his journey and I'd traveled with him as far as I could go.

Clearing out a desk drawer, I uncovered a folder with travel brochures of places we'd visited over the years. Geoff's bold script annotations in the margins diminished to a thin scrawl with the passage of time, until they stopped altogether. How long had it taken me to realize he was unable to open an envelope or write his name? I thought of the times I'd winced when he ate too slowly. I would hold the spoon and make a small sigh waiting for him to open his mouth. Did I have to throw him a sharp look when he spilled or dropped something? Did broken china or another mess to clean up warrant harsh rebuke? The moments when I'd shown impatience and irritation formed a loop of regrets I'd have given the world to rewind and erase.

It was cold comfort, but I recalled Geoff confiding that he had to live with his own regrets after Barbara died. My mother, too, had voiced remorse that she hadn't been more patient and attentive with my grandmother. My friends had spoken to me about their own perceived failings in those moments when caregiving had overwhelmed them. I wasn't alone in having these regrets and feelings of guilt.

I remembered New Year's Eve in New York, only months before Geoff passed away, when I kissed him good night and stayed with him until he fell asleep before taking a walk. I remembered the promises I made to myself that night on the cusp of a new and very uncertain year ahead. *Patience. Kindness. No regrets.*

Can we ever have no regrets? I'm inclined to think it's part of the grieving process: not wanting to let go and imagining that if one had acted differently, death could have been forestalled.

These emotional responses were not only fresh in my mind, but preserved in the laptop journal I'd begun in late 2007 under the heading "The Day Our Lives Changed Forever." I wrote daily but had not read back through past entries at all during the course of Geoff's illness. Occasionally I wrote lengthy passages in a single sitting, but often I'd write a sentence or two a couple of times a day about something I thought ought to be recorded.

Sitting in the garden with my laptop open to the file, I began reading from the beginning, realizing those passages marked the start of my grieving for a life that was slipping away. At first, I'd dutifully noted medications and shifts in behavior. Occasionally I'd added a stilted comment about my reactions to these changes, putting a good face on my response to each new setback—essentially lying about my feelings to my own journal! Owning up to what I was actually going through had just been too hard. I couldn't put on paper what would sound like bleak, self-pitying whining, not in those early stages when I was struggling to cope with the very thought that my husband had an incurable disease.

I recognized a turning point in my own form of denial in a passage I wrote about the two of us attending a memorial for a dear friend. Many of the guests were former colleagues of Geoff's, none of whom were yet aware of his recent diagnosis—and he wanted to keep it that way as long as possible. I'd taken pride in enabling the deception by surreptitiously helping Geoff move through the crowded restaurant, confidently using leverage when I had to hoist him out of a chair. We'd practiced the maneuvers at home, and I was convinced I did it so naturally and easily that nobody noticed how much assistance he needed. So sure were we that we had fooled everyone, we called it the "Fred and Ginger thing."

Unfortunately, just as we were leaving the memorial, we lost our balance and both fell over, toppling tables and chairs, sending wine-glasses and peanuts flying everywhere. People rushed to help us back onto our feet. We laughed and joked, but we were both humiliated and kept apologizing.

"Everyone saw," Geoff said as we made our way to the car. "Let's hope they think we're drunk."

"It was my fault. My feet weren't planted right. How many people do you think we soaked in red wine?"

While I accepted responsibility, I also managed to persuade him it was time to inform friends about his diagnosis. As a result, I became more comfortable expressing my emotions: as the disease progressed, my journal entries were far more raw and personal, the grief expressed painful, at times, to read.

In the final months of Geoff's life, I'd recorded a recurring dream which also became a sort of waking reverie that sometimes lulled me to sleep. I saw myself in spacious white surroundings, furnished simply, with a circular staircase and a view of mountains and ocean. In my waking moments, I added soft light and accents of crystal and silver, imagining rooms taking shape with minimal furniture in spaces devoid of clutter. There was no sign of handicap equipment. The presence of a circular staircase alone indicated this was a place where Geoff didn't reside.

Not surprisingly, the beginnings of the dream had accompanied the arrival of home hospice care. The dream unsettled me, inducing waves of guilt whenever I thought about it. Did it represent wishful thinking? Or was it a natural reaction to the oxygen tank in the closet and morphine in the vegetable crisper, evidence that the end was near and I'd soon be on my own? I wrote about it in my journal, but at the time could not confide that dream to anyone.

Some time later, widows and widowers I met in a grief group mentioned similar dreams and the guilt induced by imagining life without a loved one. I was encouraged to accept it as a natural reaction—described by a friend, who was both a widow and a psychologist, as "an instinctive survival response in a time of emotional trauma." Those were fancy words for feelings so nakedly raw and guilt inducing, yet comforting to hear.

But sitting in my garden, reading those passages, I felt very alone. How would I handle a future on my own? I realized I had no interest in relocating to the spacious white habitat with a circular staircase, decorated in accents of crystal and silver, however enticing it had appeared in my dreams. I liked my home and wanted to be surrounded by familiar furnishings and warm memories of Geoff.

Chapter Ten

I spent Easter weekend with friends at their beach house, writing in my journal: Easter morning . . . I awaken early, not quite six o'clock. It's drizzling outside, the beach and sky a unified gray. I make coffee. It's silent except for the cawing of birds and steady wash of ocean on the beach. I discover a piece I wrote has been published in the London *Sunday Telegraph*, and I read it online. It's beautifully edited, and that brings on a fresh flood of tears. Geoff would have loved reading it.

I walk on the beach, thinking about Geoff, of course. I walk perhaps a mile, not quite realizing that I'm both talking to Geoff and about him. In that time, the remembrance forms in my thoughts. I know what I will say at his memorial. Of course I'll do the eulogy—how else will I make it through the service? As I near the house, my cell phone rings. It's an old friend, a widower himself. "Sundays are the hardest," he tells me . . .

On Tuesday I meet with Father Gabri to plan the memorial service. He'll ask me who will do the remembrance, and I'll tell him I will, wondering if he thinks that's odd and if I can handle it. All he's seen me do is cry.

The week of reflection was restorative, giving me fresh perspective. Rested and feeling stronger emotionally, I knew it was time to get on with living. With holidays over, my friend Bridget drove me to the mortuary. I'd packed up Geoff's best suit, shoes, Turnbull & Asser shirt bought in

London, his favorite tie I'd given him, and newly purchased underwear and socks. I might have thought I was now fully prepared to make decisions, but whatever the funeral director said to me, I seemed to hear through a fog. Luckily, Bridget took notes and jumped in when I was about to accept terms she knew I'd regret. At the same time, she reminded me of things I needed to ask about, such as the particular wording on the headstone. Afterward, my sterling advocate took me for a fancy brunch—and yes, I recommend libation accompanying eggs after a trip to a mortuary.

I soon had plans in place for the funeral, a graveside service with family and close friends attending. Everything was organized for the memorial service that would be held at the church the following day, with Father Gabri officiating and many more people expected. A caterer friend was preparing the memorial luncheon at my women's club. My book-club friends were providing desserts. What had I overlooked that still needed doing? I checked my reminder list for calls still to be made and arrangements to finalize, but everything that needed doing had been done. Why did it seem I had so much time on my hands? I had many offers of help, but if anyone helped me, I would have had even less to do!

As always, I awakened early. But instead of immediately tending to Geoff, I lay in bed thinking about him, missing him, and weeping. I felt empty without him beside me, my life lacking purpose in his absence. I no longer had a routine to follow or caregiving tasks to occupy my time. Everything was too easy, too unencumbered. I moved quickly, doing things so swiftly and efficiently that I was left with empty hands, feeling useless. I made coffee and puttered in the garden, my day's to-do list blank. I knew I should be doing something, but I couldn't think what. I'd been a caregiver and a wife, and now I was neither. On forms, I had to check a box marked "widow," but it wasn't a role I knew how to play—or even comprehend. What did a widow do? I filled an empty afternoon by baking oatmeal cookies, Geoff's favorite.

❖　❖　❖

Bridget offered to pick me up early on the morning of the graveside funeral so I could have time alone with Geoff at the mortuary before friends and family arrived, some driving to the cemetery directly from the airport. Wearing a twelve-year-old black pantsuit Geoff bought for me in Paris, I stood with an armload of fresh flowers from the garden. There would be many beautiful flower tributes, but for his gravesite I wanted a mixed bouquet of the roses, freesia and calla lilies Geoff loved seeing in our garden.

I entered the silent viewing room on my own, approaching the casket shyly. I hadn't seen Geoff in over two weeks, and he didn't look as I remembered him, his face uncharacteristically stern. I reminded myself that he'd had a full autopsy, his brain dispatched to a medical research lab. Why would he look like himself? I'd provided the mortuary with his best business suit, but the attire now struck me as inappropriate for his final journey—he ought to be wearing his preferred traveling attire, his safari jacket and blue jeans. Did he see my disappointment? I touched his forehead, my mind superimposing an image of the once strong, vital man with merry eyes and sunny smile I knew as Geoff, my husband.

I was sure the good-looking Irish priest included in the Holy Cross mortuary package moonlighted as an actor. Perhaps channeling Bing Crosby, buried in a nearby plot, the priest spoke in a folksy, mellifluous brogue as though he and Geoff had been lifelong pub mates. On such a somber occasion, his warmth induced smiles along with the tears and penetrating sadness that the flesh-and-blood man, who loved a good story and a pint among friends, would no longer be part of our lives.

While everyone congregated at the gravesite after the service, I stepped to the side to answer my cell phone—and wished I hadn't. A representative from a credit card company told me they'd been informed the primary person on a joint account had died, and the card had been canceled. Charges for funeral expenses on that card had been denied. Of all the things to have to concern myself with during my husband's funeral, this struck me as diabolical. But it was also a reminder of the real-life issues I would be handling on my own and the myriad phone calls and business matters still to be dealt with in the coming days.

After the funeral, family and friends ate lunch sitting around the long table in the garden, telling stories and reminiscing about Geoff. The setting was tranquil, with the gentle splashing of the fountain on the ivy-covered wall and the sweet scent of roses in full bloom. By midafternoon, family members were engaged in what Norwegians tend to do for leisure: making themselves useful. Instead of napping, reading or sunbathing by the pool, everyone changed into jeans and T-shirts to scour the house for odd jobs to do.

My younger brother, David, who is blind, stood listening to the splash of the fountain, then announced exactly why it was leaking. He fixed it, an ordinary task for a man who does fine cabinetry work and built his own log cabin by hand on a remote island in Lake Superior. My other brother and nephew disassembled the railings and motorized chair installed on the stairs for Geoff's safety, encasing the heavy, cumbersome apparatus in sheets of plastic to store in the garage. My sisters-in-law and niece gave me a hand in the kitchen.

If they hadn't all pitched in to help me, we wouldn't have discovered boxes of sound recordings stored in a space behind the stairs since long before Geoff and I married. I had no idea the cartons were there, and I'm sure Geoff had forgotten about them. Among vintage jazz records, we uncovered a collection of homemade acetate recordings and reel-to-reel tapes dating back to Geoff's childhood. What a shame I hadn't found these boxes earlier so Geoff and I could have listened to these treasures together. He'd made one of them at age twelve, recording his brother and parents, all since deceased, talking together at the dinner table on Christmas Eve. How charming to hear his mother, whom I had never met, speculate whether Bing or Ol' Blue Eyes might sing a solo with the choir at midnight mass. His father, who had passed away the year Geoff started the magazine, spoke in the same rolling baritone as his son. What a precious gift to eavesdrop on a joyful celebration among family members I wish I could have known.

Close friends joined my family for dinner, cooked on the grill in the upper garden. It was a warm evening, but as the air grew cool and damp, I suggested everyone go into Geoff's closet to find something warm to wear. While wearing his jackets, sweaters, shirts, scarves and hats, we all sat around the table reminiscing about Geoff, recalling our many other evenings together under the stars. That night, I urged everyone to take whatever they'd found in his closet home with them and return again and again wearing his clothes.

The following day I gave the eulogy at the memorial service and greeted the many friends attending the reception at the Beverly Hills Women's Club. Afterward, the last of my family members departed, and I looked around my quiet, empty house. The living room was fragrant with floral arrangements, the refrigerator stocked with gifts of food. Thanks to my family, there was no sign of the stair lift, the fountain didn't leak and there were no squeaky doorknobs or loose hinges. My sisters-in-law had made sure my Tupperware drawer was a thing of beauty and efficiency, every cupboard orderly.

Good friends had helped empty Geoff's closet and would return for dinners in the garden wearing his jackets, sweaters and scarves. Candelaria had done the rest, helping me pack up clothing for donation to the homeless program at church—but leaving his tattered safari jacket still hanging in the coat closet, a reminder he'd left without it and wouldn't be returning. I walked through the silent house, realizing what a gift they had all given me, each in their own way assisting me in this transition to daily life without Geoff.

Chapter Eleven

The attorney who had assisted us with estate planning called to offer her condolences and ask if I needed any help. I thanked her for getting in touch and, feeling a bit smug, told her I'd handled everything on my own. I assured her that, with so much time on my hands, I'd already made all the necessary calls regarding business and estate matters.

"Oh, no," she said quickly, before I could say goodbye. "You've only just begun." I listened grimly as she rattled off everything else I needed to do. "But don't worry about overlooking anything. I'll send you some documents and email a list of what's still to be done."

I hate filling out forms, and numbers are not my friends. I slogged through a deluge of paperwork that I referred to as "widow work," wondering why everyone in the world seemed to need a copy of his death certificate, then ordered more. But in a phone call to inform one party that my husband had died, I had to laugh when a hapless clerk blurted, "Great, I know how to handle that!" I told her I could use some advice.

I found myself spending long hours in Geoff's study, sitting at his desk, spinning his Rolodex and rummaging through files for necessary documents, occasionally horrified by the thought that vital papers had almost been thrown away. Still, I sensed his wary eyes on me as I opened drawers and gingerly rifled through the remaining contents, something I would never have considered doing in his lifetime. Even when he became too infirm to open mail and I took over handling our financial and business matters, I'd still been respectful of his desk. I'm neat; he wasn't, but I was mindful not to try to bring my sense of order to his clutter.

One day, working with Geoff at his desk, I'd made my way to the bottom of a stack of mail and said, "Oh, look, wood!"

He gave me a look that said my quip was not appreciated. In the "guy universe," I realized, a man's desk is inviolate.

But when I wasn't completing those necessary tasks, I found I had an abundance of leisure that was far more burdensome than being too busy. I did not know how to occupy the buckets of unstructured free time in the void where caregiving had been. I'd pick up a book and put it down again, feeling guilty that I was indulging myself and not being *useful*. I should be *doing* something.

Friends and family were attentive. I knew from my own experience how difficult it is to make those calls to the newly bereaved, wanting to find the right words to express comfort and solace. I was well aware that my grief in losing Geoff was shared by friends, family and former colleagues who also missed having him in their lives. I made sure to offer them comforting words in return.

I recently read a piece written by a former colleague of Geoff's in which she expresses the hurt and frustration she experienced in the aftermath of her husband's death. Some friends, she wrote, were more interested in the effect of his death on themselves than on her, a narcissism she found particularly painful when a friend, expressing her utter devastation at the husband's death, said, "It must be hard on you, too."

During the time after Geoff's funeral, I was often struck by statements I knew were genuine, heartfelt words of condolence, but poorly expressed. A friend I'm very fond of told me that her dog died the week Geoff passed away, "so I really know how you feel." I was taken aback, but I understood what she meant, knowing she was desolated by the loss of her beloved pet.

What made me cringe, though, was hearing someone tell me, "Geoff is in a far, far better place." *No, he's not!* I wanted to shout. *His place is with me, which would be far, far better!*

Or, "After all you've been through, it must be a relief that it's over." *No, I don't want it over! I want him back, no matter what!*

Or, "You have your memories to bring you comfort." *Yes, and the terrible ache that we can't make more memories together!*

The truth is, losing a loved one is a lousy, miserable experience. "I'm so sorry," says it all.

But for each well-meaning but regrettable remark, I received scores of well-composed, artfully written personal tributes to my husband for having nurtured, befriended and encouraged a multitude of writers and young interns. Many of the letters were from people I'd never met, including a distinguished newspaper editor in the Midwest who wrote movingly about Geoff reaching out and mentoring him through a rough patch early in his career. I learned about my husband's many acts of kindness, fellowship and caring, knowing only too well what a gift he'd been in my own life. I wrote personal notes in longhand, spending considerable time over each one, thanking the many people who had sent flowers and condolence cards.

Aside from handling the business end of fresh widowhood, I was having difficulty refocusing on myself, both personally and professionally. I wanted to get back to work writing and acting, which meant getting in touch with my agents to set the wheels in motion. The void in my social life was less easily managed. I'd dropped out of so much in order to be available for Geoff, yet resuming some of those activities didn't feel appropriate, either. Reinstating lapsed memberships and picking up the strands of projects I'd abandoned felt like taking steps backward just to fill time. My life was very changed, and so was I. Even as I mulled what my future could hold, I thought of Jane's exhortation that life is not a dress rehearsal—get on with it!

❖   ❖   ❖

At the end of each day I dealt with an obligatory function I preferred to avoid: feeding myself. I rarely entered the kitchen after my early morning coffee, but I knew I had to deal with nourishment at least once a day. Part of the reason I avoided cooking was that meals and their preparation had played a significant role in my life with Geoff. He arose even earlier than me and always delivered a tray with coffee, fruit and toast to our bedroom with the morning newspapers. We enjoyed grocery shopping together, especially at neighborhood farmers markets and artisanal shops, and I loved having him keep me company in the kitchen while I prepared meals. Geoff wasn't a cook, but he excelled at setting the scene with candlelight, music and good wine. Often we'd dine in the garden under a starlit sky, with a crackling fire in the outdoor fireplace, and talk late into the evening.

Aside from missing our wonderful mealtimes together, I discovered that buying food for one person, preparing single portions and dining alone is just not fun. Thawing out ready-made meals was particularly unappealing. I did not relish eating by myself while watching the evening news. I knew I'd eventually get the hang of it, but I just wasn't up to the effort of making myself a meal. Nor, I realized, was I prone to leaving the house other than for a combined trip to the bank, post office and gym. Life on my own was proving to be not unlike the days I spent as a full-time caregiver.

For the better part of several years, I'd essentially been housebound. I'd grown used to a routine—early to bed, early to rise, and days largely spent fulfilling Geoff's needs. I felt safe at home. I could cry whenever I felt like it. Life did not require mascara and lipstick, or even shoes.

My trips to the outside world became a walk in the garden or a swim in the pool. I realized how lucky I was that I could mourn in private, but a steady diet of it, without much food involved, was becoming unhealthy. I was a step away from eating scrambled egg out of a skillet over the sink when it occurred to me that Happy Hour was the answer.

The concept of Happy Hour had served us well when Geoff was ill: a sociable time in the late afternoon when we could gather with friends at home—and yes, eat. It was something to look forward to, a break from too much enforced togetherness. Friends brought laughter and good conversation, relieving our isolation. With Geoff gone, I no longer had an excuse to close myself off—and I had every reason to rejoin the outside world. If a convivial atmosphere in which to enjoy good food and drink at sundown can be considered therapeutic, Happy Hour fit the bill.

I instituted a new routine, going for a long walk in the late afternoon and then heading to one of the neighborhood restaurants Geoff and I had once enjoyed for their Happy Hour menu. I scoured the Internet for recommendations, finding upscale steak houses with piano bars (petit filet and pinot noir), Mexican cantinas (quesadillas and margaritas), French bistros (quiche and Beaujolais), Italian trattorias (calamari and pinot grigio) and, always my favorite, hamburger joints serving sliders and French fries with the house merlot. I relished having such wide choices, often exploring unfamiliar neighborhoods in search of a new place I'd found online.

Soon pals were teasing me about my lengthy roster of Happy Hour venues and joining me for the novelty of trying new places. The spontaneity of meeting a friend for Happy Hour took the pressure off sitting through a lengthy dinner I didn't feel up to enjoying. I could also drop in to a restaurant at Happy Hour and, surrounded by other singles, not feel out of place on my own. I didn't bring a book or otherwise engage myself, which left me open to responding to people around me. Not having to plan or make a reservation suited me, giving me the freedom to navigate my rocky emotional terrain at my own speed.

Happy Hour get-togethers became my social world, possibly the most positive new addition to my life. Friends were good about the tears. Unexpectedly, whatever the time or circumstance, my voice would catch and my eyes puddle with a flood of tears; I seemed to have no control over them. I'd also find any excuse to mention Geoff's name in conversation. I'd had enough experience with grieving friends to know these were natural occurrences for someone dealing with fresh loss. I didn't hold back when a wave of emotion overcame me, but neither did I want to wear out friends with prolonged shows of grief.

In time, I knew the desire to speak Geoff's name aloud, as though keeping him alive and present, would recede and the tears become less constant. Until then, I trusted friends understood and would stand by me in this phase of grieving.

Chapter Twelve

I stayed close to home in the months following Geoff's death, but I sensed him hovering, pulling strings and steering me back into work, travel and fully engaging with the world again. If not for some divine intervention, how else could I account for the abundance of writing and acting work coming my way—and the opportunity to return to London? After considerable delay, *Dark Shadows*, the television series that launched my career, was being given its third silver-screen incarnation thanks to two of its devoted fans, Tim Burton and Johnny Depp. Could the actor who made Jack Sparrow part of a multibillion-dollar franchise do the same playing Barnabas Collins? That was the hope as four of us—stars from the original television series and the two previous feature films—flew to England in June to play cameos in the Warner Bros. production.

Jonathan Frid (Barnabas Collins), Lara Parker (Angelique Bouchard), David Selby (Quentin Collins) and I (Josette du Pres and Maggie Evans) delighted in working together again, albeit on the periphery of an extravagant production we could not for the world have imagined when we did the original series. On our first day at Pinewood Studios, we toured the back lot, where the town of Collinsport had been recreated, with shop fronts lining cobblestone streets and fishing boats bobbing in a harbor constructed in a mammoth tank of water. On the spectacular interior set of the Collinwood mansion, Jonathan Frid confronted his doppelganger, Johnny Depp, in makeup and costume as Barnabas Collins, and scrutinized him closely. "I see you've done the hair," Jonathan noted, studying the spiky forelocks he'd introduced some forty-five years earlier.

"We're doing things a little differently," Johnny replied, quickly chorusing with director Tim Burton, "But we wouldn't be here without you."

It was a bittersweet journey in every respect. If the film hadn't been delayed, I would not have been able to leave Geoff to work in England—and if the film had been postponed much longer, Jonathan, who was elderly and showing signs of frailty, might not have been well enough to make the trip. For the granddaddy of contemporary vampires, his cameo in this camped-up resurrection of the series he'd made famous would mark his final appearance on camera. Jonathan passed away before the film's premiere in May 2012.

The trip also provided an opportunity to return to the Cottage for a final visit. Our stays in London had grown less frequent with Geoff's illness. Ben, too, rarely made the trip, and we'd jointly made the wrenching decision to give up our treasured London Cottage. On the afternoon I stopped by, workmen were busy gutting the 1791 structure, combining two bedrooms to create one with an en suite bathroom that would not have a vintage pull-chain toilet or deep claw-foot bathtub. Evidence of the dismantling was piled in the courtyard, including kitchen cupboards I'd refinished myself and the handrail for the perilous staircase Geoff had had difficulty climbing. I peered inside and wished I hadn't. The stark interior, missing its fireplace and beamed ceiling, bore little resemblance to my cozy home of nearly forty years. I missed her and all she'd meant to me. I heard the ripping of walls on the second floor and felt her pain. It was mine.

After two weeks in London, I flew home to Los Angeles, arriving in the early afternoon. I was tired after the long flight but went straight to my garden, flourishing with hydrangea, lilies and roses. I filled a basket then left for the cemetery to visit Geoff, impulsively pocketing a small photo album off the piano on my way out the door.

Driving to the cemetery that afternoon, I thought of a clinical psychologist friend who knew of my frequent visits to the gravesite. He'd startled me one evening over dinner by asking, "You don't really think he's *there*, do you?"

His tone—which I perceived as scoffing—seemed intended to mock my faith as well as my sanity. I explained, as if to a child, that no, I did not think Geoff was really *there* since bits and pieces of him had been harvested for donor transplant and medical research. The cemetery represented the last place I'd physically left him, and his grave provided me with a place of significance where I could sit and reflect on our life together.

"Do you talk to him?" my friend persisted.

"I talk to myself as much as to the Geoff I knew and loved."

I didn't mention the spiritual connection to Geoff that I experienced in that tranquil setting with trees, grass and expanse of sky, or admit that I did speak directly to him, pouring my heart out. Who else could I confide in? Only Geoff would understand that the Cottage, my home for much of my adult life, had its own spiritual significance to me. The Cottage had also figured in our romantic getaways over the years, making our frequent travels abroad convenient and affordable, and he would share my grief at that era's passing.

I thought about the peace and comfort that drew me to the cemetery as I walked across the dewy grass along a parade of gravestones, all uniform in size and shape, but each having shifted, settled and aged with the passage of time. Geoff's headstone, the newest among them, was also sinking into the sod, skewing sideways and taking on its own weathered mottling.

The turf on his grave was thick and smooth, the earth healing far more quickly than I was. I knelt on a straw mat and arranged the flowers, then buried my face in the perfumed mass, feeling so raw and torn I could barely breathe. *Too soon! Come back!*

"It's foolish of me, I know," I told the bristly grass covering his grave. "But just give me a moment when I feel we're together again the way we once were."

I flipped open the scrapbook, feeling a thump of pleasure seeing a snapshot of Geoff taken on our honeymoon in Paris, his hair dark and curly. He looked handsome and carefree. Why didn't this youthful image spring to mind when I thought of him, rather than how he had been as he lay dying at the tail end of all our years together? Here he was on the pages of the album enjoying picnics, hikes, dinners in the garden and travel in faraway places—that's how I wanted to remember him, without snapshots to remind me. I longed to picture Geoff striding toward me, radiating warmth and happiness in his blue jeans and safari jacket, which would always hang in our coat closet. I glanced at another photograph of us at a gala premiere—posing together on a red carpet, smiling and holding hands amidst the starry frenzy swirling around us, and knowing we'd be going home together.

I gazed longest at a favorite photo I'd snapped in our garden of Geoff wearing an old T-shirt, stubble of a beard hollowing his cheeks, a martini poised in his hand. I'd captured a look in his eyes so intimate— that held such love and longing—it made me blush at the memory of putting down the camera and leaning in for a kiss.

A chill breeze swept across my shoulders. Night was falling.

"Let's go home." I picked up my belongings and walked toward my car, calling over my shoulder, "C'mon, Geoff. It's getting late. Come home with me."

If that meant I was nuts, I'd live with it.

I'd grown close to Dr. Yvette Bordelon, Geoff's neurologist, who stopped by the house for coffee one afternoon, bringing copies of the autopsy reports. I read the documents dry-eyed, grateful to have Yvette on hand to offer clarifications. In clear clinical terms, the documents provided postmortem confirmation of Geoff's diagnosis: progressive supranuclear palsy. The reports left no doubt that the outcome of Geoff's disease had been inevitable. Nothing could have been done to turn the verdict around or extend his life. I also learned that in the phase II clinical trial he'd participated in, Geoff had been taking the full dosage of the experimental drug, not a placebo. It was time to stop second-guessing and accept that we'd tried everything we could.

It was also time to deal with my own medical issues. During Geoff's illness, I'd postponed or canceled various doctor appointments, either because something came up at the last minute or I just couldn't find the time to sit in a doctor's waiting room. The primary ailment was my right hip, which required joint replacement. Assisting Geoff, particularly transferring him into the car and loading the wheelchair in the trunk, had taken its toll. Each step was painful. I'd begun dragging my leg and had trouble lassoing my toes with a sock.

I required cataract surgery and had neglected making appointments for a mammogram, colonoscopy, dermatology screening and dental checkups. I imagined finding some big-box department-store version of a medical facility where I could just drop in and say, "Please, check me out and fix me." Even my car was long overdue for a tune-up. Putting off caring for my own needs, I soon discovered, was not unusual among caregivers.

Those needs were not only physical. A close friend who was a recent widow herself suggested I join a grief group. "Talking with other people who have suffered recent loss will help you adjust," she said. "It's time."

I'd convinced myself I was adjusting quite well on my own, and I was resistant to sharing my personal feelings with complete strangers.

However, after continued urging, I reluctantly signed up for a support group. I arrived early for the first Monday-afternoon session and pulled into a parking space directly in front of the entrance to the building.

For long minutes I sat in the car, engine running, trying to convince myself to attend the meeting. I watched several people arrive who I guessed were among my peer group ("seniors fifty-plus who have lost spouses"), and they all looked as grim as I felt. Did I really want to hear their struggles with grief—or share mine? I was mortified at the thought I might break down weeping in front of everyone. Having a root canal struck me as a less torturous way to spend an hour, but then I questioned my hostile reaction to the meeting. Did it emanate from fear of probing my own feelings? If others in the same boat could face attending this grief group session, so would I. I put money in the meter and went inside.

We were four widows, three widowers and a grief counselor named Carol sitting in a cluster of mismatched chairs around a coffee table with a candy bowl and boxes of tissues. I was last to arrive and plunged my hand into the candy bowl, my heart beating wildly at the prospect of having to even speak my name. When it was my turn to introduce myself, I burst into tears. I was not the only one. We were roughly the same age but came from various ethnic, religious and economic backgrounds, with seemingly little in common other than mourning the recent deaths of spouses. By the time we got through introductions, I realized we had a good deal in common in addition to struggling with grief.

Sharing feelings of sorrow and emotional distress in a group setting, with a moderator guiding us through sticky patches, turned out to be therapeutic and comforting. Instead of being embarrassed about my tearful meltdown, I felt release. I opened up about feelings of anger, guilt and regret that I would not have mentioned to even a close friend, but could in this protected environment. We followed protocol and didn't make direct inquiries or give unsolicited advice, but we each spoke to the group as a whole. We were gentle and respectful with each other. Despite being provided with a list of everyone's name and contact information, our confidences felt contained and protected by mutual empathy. We were no longer strangers to each other.

It was beneficial to learn I was not the only one dragging a leg or having trouble putting socks on. Another woman was on crutches, recovering from a broken ankle. A man had a bandaged hand, having burned it while preparing a meal. Someone else had dislocated a shoulder in a fall. Everyone spoke of recent mishaps, injuries and "seeming to be more prone to accidents."

A woman mentioned feeling "more vulnerable physically," and we nodded agreement.

"I think twice before getting on a ladder now that I'm on my own," a man said.

Most, like me, were dealing with a backlog of medical and dental appointments "there just hadn't been time for before."

"Losing things" was another common refrain.

In fact, rummaging through my handbag after the session, I couldn't find my car keys. They weren't in my pocket, nor had I dropped them on the floor. I looked everywhere. Dismayed, I returned to my car hoping I'd find my keys on the sidewalk.

It was then that I noticed my car window was partially open and jazz was playing on the radio. My keys were on the passenger seat. I'd left my Prius unlocked, the engine running the entire time I was in the session.

After that clear sign I could use a bit more help adjusting, I continued to attend the grief group sessions. Among the subjects we discussed in our weekly meetings were positive things we'd introduced to our lives—and I mentioned Happy Hour. At the group's request, the following session I handed out a list of my favorite restaurants that offered Happy Hour, complete with addresses and sample bar menus.

The next day, one of the men in the group called to ask if I'd like to get together with him for Happy Hour. I said, "Sure, where would you like to meet?"

"I've already made a reservation," he said. "I'll pick you up at eight o'clock."

"No," I blurted, panic rising. "Happy Hour is five to seven o'clock. No reservations. I'll just meet you somewhere."

"It's no trouble. I'll pick you up, and we'll make eight o'clock happy!"

"Okay," I stammered. Displaying the social ineptness of a backward thirteen-year-old, I'd managed to commit myself to what sounded like a date—whoops!

He was a very nice man, couldn't have been nicer, but the last thing I had in mind was going on a date with *anyone*. The idea of going out as a *couple*—stumbling politely through that awkward getting-to-know-someone-new phase—made me quake. I saw myself bolting before the appetizers arrived.

But it's just a *meal*, not a prom date, my sensible self said. *One* meal, so what's the big deal? My less reasonable self resisted, my stomach taking an elevator ride at the very thought of the upcoming ordeal, but having accepted his invitation, I couldn't think how to get out of it.

Only months into mourning, going on a date felt like a huge betrayal of my husband. I was still wrestling with the concept of widowhood and couldn't even bear referring to myself as a widow. I wore a wedding ring and considered myself married—except that my husband had died. Whatever the nature of the illusion I clung to, I wasn't inclined to alter it. I continued to say "we" and "our," as I always had, with Geoff's name rising to my lips at every opportunity.

I remembered Geoff telling me that after Barbara died, he'd immediately gotten invitations to dinner parties to "fill out the table." After years of nursing an invalid wife, friends and colleagues tried to swiftly ease him back into a couples social world. He'd had no end of invitations from hostesses eager to match him up, and phone calls from women with "an extra ticket" to an event or an occasion that required an escort.

In truth, rather than "filling out the table," I was more often the extra woman among couples at the few dinner parties I attended. I couldn't imagine myself becoming the gal with "an extra ticket" and calling around for an escort. Frankly, I felt less discomfort venturing out on my own than in attempting to wrangle a companion. I'd already walked one red carpet alone and knew I'd do so again.

When eight o'clock rolled around that evening, I dreaded hearing the doorbell—*why hadn't I insisted on meeting at the restaurant?* I opened the door to find my grief group friend nattily dressed with an armload of red roses, which meant inviting him in while I found a vase. Dinner was several courses at a restaurant too posh for Happy Hour and established with unmistakable certainty that I was being wooed. I clutched my handbag in my lap and tried to behave like a grown-up. But instead of the evening turning into the uncomfortable encounter I'd feared, we ended up having a lively conversation about romance—he was up for it, I was not.

He made his intentions toward me clear. I warmly thanked him for making all the right romantic gestures but let him know I wasn't ready to date *anyone*, that the idea hadn't even crossed my mind. He'd already signed up for an online dating service and was eager to embrace a new relationship. More than that, he saw himself marrying again, "as soon as I find the right woman." His wife, he told me, had encouraged him to find a new mate once she was gone. "She knew I wouldn't be any good on my own."

Once he'd reconciled himself to the fact that I wasn't a girlfriend candidate, we spoke freely about what it was like living alone. He'd nursed a wife he loved through a long illness and couldn't bear the emptiness and solitude now that she was gone. "I hate the loneliness," he confided, "and not having someone to just be with." His adult children, mourning the fairly recent loss of their mother, were not thrilled that he was dating, "but they don't know what it's like walking into a dark, silent house and being completely alone."

That night, when he dropped me off at home, I entered a dark, silent house and felt very alone. But even though he'd cajoled me into saying that someday I might be open to a new relationship, I couldn't even imagine it. In the meantime, I fixed him up with a close friend who was single and very much looking for romance.

Chapter Thirteen

The first year after losing a loved one is fraught with reminders, a calendar full of holidays and family occasions to face alone. Each day seemed to present a new milestone, yet another experience that wouldn't include Geoff. As close as I am to my brothers, a boisterous traditional Christmas celebration with family was more than I thought I could handle. Nor did I want to dampen their festivities, my presence alone a reminder to them of Geoff's absence from our lives.

I returned to our apartment in New York to spend the holidays on my own, wanting nothing more than the comfort of familiar surroundings. I opened the door and glanced at the couch, struck at not finding Geoff sitting there waiting for me, a smile lighting his face as he looked up to see me. *You should be here!* I told the vacant sofa. I plopped down on the cushion next to where he always sat, my hand stretching across the empty space, sensing his presence in the stillness.

Get used to this, I told myself. *This is the way it is.*

Yet change of any sort upset me. While I had to get used to missing Geoff, I wanted everything else in my world to remain the same. I'd rage at the least sign that something was missing or not as it had been. During a walk through my neighborhood, I stopped in front of a gaping hole in the earth where a crane was demolishing the last of an old building Geoff and I had loved for its quaint front stoop and oak-beamed coffee house. I keenly felt its loss, knowing a high-rise he would never see would be erected in its place.

I went to church and was dismayed that wooden pews, well over a century old and worn to a lustrous patina, had been replaced with interlocking cushioned chairs. *Chairs!* I swallowed hard and sat down, wondering if God was as displeased as I was.

I drew comfort from the familiar local shops, buying a poinsettia from the corner florist and whole-grain bread from a nearby bakery while ignoring the fancy new market that had opened a few blocks away. I walked along the river, sitting on the same bench where, as a student new to New York decades earlier, I'd written letters home to my family on warm Sunday afternoons. Bundled up against the cold, I'd brought Geoff there in his wheelchair on a sunny winter day only a year earlier.

How odd to be walking the streets of New York *not* pushing a wheelchair. I still fixated on curbs, avoiding the ones cracked or pooled in water, and chose sidewalks that were wide and smooth. Without thinking twice, I leaped up to help a man secure his wheelchair in position on the bus and helped a woman using a walker board the lift. Geoff had gotten a kick out of riding the wheelchair lift. On one occasion, the bus was so crowded that after locking his chair in place, I sat on Geoff's lap and gave him a kiss, prompting smiles from passengers standing around us.

Unable to shake my sadness on New Year's Eve, I went to bed well before midnight and had a vivid dream in which I was standing amid a pile of luggage in a vast hotel lobby, looking around for a bellhop. I left my red handbag on top of the luggage because I wasn't able to assist Geoff and also carry my handbag—yet I knew I shouldn't leave it, because someone could snatch it.

I treasured the red handbag Geoff had bought me in Italy, and it was showing wear because I used it so often. I turned back, warning myself to hang it on my arm for safety—but it was gone! I looked around the huge, crowded lobby for the bag, but I couldn't keep searching, because Geoff needed me and was waiting for me.

The booming sound of fireworks woke me at midnight. I got out of bed and checked on my handbag, safe where I'd left it on a chair by the front door. I pulled a warm coat on over my nightie and stepped into boots to walk down the street to the same spot on the East River where I'd stood a year earlier after putting Geoff to bed. Fireworks pounded in the distance, and the night sky glowed with splashes of brilliant light erupting behind bridges and tall buildings.

Somewhere close by, likely from a party in the River House across the street, I heard the tinkling sounds of a piano. Swaying to the music and humming a familiar melody, I imagined leaning into Geoff, feeling the warmth of his hands on my arms. The lingering memory of being in his embrace only reminded me of how much I yearned for the real thing, but at least I could picture the laughter and mischief in his eyes as he pulled me close. It would have to do.

Chapter Fourteen

Appropriately enough, on New Year's Day I took a long walk and thought ahead to how I would make the most of the coming year. My pace brisk, I traversed snow-lined paths in Central Park ticking off a mental list of priorities. High on the agenda was promotion of my first novel, which would be published in August. I'd written much of it on my laptop while sitting next to Geoff as he dozed or watched television. When I'd finished the first draft of *Dark Passages*, a humorous paranormal romance, I read the entire manuscript aloud to him, pausing to note his comments in the margins.

"I hope you realize you've written about your mother," he'd said. Really? A story about mother and daughter vampires who didn't quite get along? I'd laughed, appreciating his insight. How would I ever manage without my superb in-house editor and first reader?

Other projects kept me busy, too. I was looking forward to the premiere of Tim Burton's *Dark Shadows* film, hoping the movie and our brief cameo appearances would rise to expectations. My agents knew that after a lengthy hiatus as a caregiver, I was ready to go back to work acting. I'd already enrolled in an acting class taught by a beloved teacher I'd studied with at the beginning of my career. Acting and writing had always been my twin pursuits, and I was excited about fully engaging in both again. I didn't think of myself as picking up the pieces of my active life before Geoff became ill; rather, I saw myself as starting fresh, expanding my horizons with new ventures.

As it should be, I thought, recalling Jane's admonishment to me decades earlier: *Live life fully; don't waste a precious moment of it.* She had always urged me to push the boundaries and take on new challenges. "After all," she said, "we come into this world alone and leave it alone . . . we must aim high and become the best of ourselves."

It wasn't only Jane's words that guided me. I also thought of my mother, who confided one afternoon that she'd found the time spent living on her own after my father passed away to be some of the most satisfying and enjoyable years of her life. I laughed, chiding her that I'd hoped to hear raising children and looking after my father had brought her the most pleasure. She gave me a look, which made me laugh even more.

Jesting aside, I understood what she was telling me. My mother had been born during World War I, graduated from school during the Great Depression, married, bore children and lived as a farm wife during World War II. She'd spent much of her life in service to others, working full-time and devoting herself to church, community and all the pressing concerns of family life. She'd nursed my father through a long illness when he'd been unable to work, and attended to the special medical needs of two of her children. After fifty-four years of a close and loving marriage, my father passed away.

My mother was facing her own mortality, knowing she had only weeks left to live, when she confided her feelings to me about living life on her own. We'd spent the afternoon visiting my younger sister, who is profoundly mentally retarded as a result of an Rh-negative blood factor untreated at birth. Sandra, who is unable to speak and has little cognitive ability, is well cared for in a group home where she's lived for many years. That day, my sister seemed unusually receptive to us. My mother held her hand, fed her bits of chocolate we'd brought and hugged her goodbye for the final time. On our drive home, my mother said, "You'll look after her, won't you?" I assured her I would. I'd long ago signed guardianship papers for my sister in the event of my mother's death.

But even as my mother secured my sister's care in a farewell visit, part of this tidying-up stage at the end of her life, she was also looking ahead to the next item on her agenda—passing her driver's test. At age ninety-two, her driver's license was due for renewal. "I don't s'pose I'll be driving much anymore," she said, "but I want to see if I can pass the test." She did.

It wasn't surprising behavior for a woman who, well into her so-called retirement years, continued to seek personal fulfillment by serving on the board of a Norwegian cultural organization, teaching a pastry class, volunteering in a literacy program, writing newsletter articles and learning computer skills. She liked to work and was always on the look-out for jobs that would give her a chance to meet people. In her mid-eighties, while getting her hearing aid adjusted at a nearby mall, she'd asked the manager if he needed someone to answer phones and greet people—she got the job. She liked nothing better than putting on a nice outfit with good shoes to go out in the world and feel useful.

If she'd discovered newfound purpose and gratification in the years on her own, I would let it be an inspiration to me to expand my own horizons.

Having fully recovered from both hip-replacement and cataract surgery, I looked forward to doing some traveling. In particular, I wanted to be as far away as possible in mid-April, the first anniversary of Geoff's death. I knew if I stayed at home, I would be keeping vigil, every ticking minute a countdown to his passing. China seemed like a good idea, an exotic destination I'd longed to visit and one that had not been on Geoff's travel agenda. There would be no reminders of a trip not taken, a dream not fulfilled in his lifetime. My friend Suzanne, an attorney who had recently retired, enthusiastically agreed to join me on the trip.

Together we got in touch with a travel agent and began looking at various tours. Eventually we chose Viking River Cruises, settling on the Imperial Jewels of China itinerary from Beijing to Shanghai, which included stopovers of several days in Guilin and Hong Kong before our return flight to Los Angeles. We would depart April 3 and arrive back home April 20, 2012. We booked the trip and marked our calendars. I would be in Shanghai April 16, the anniversary of Geoff's passing.

As a variously attributed adage reminds us, *Life is what happens to you while you're busy making other plans.* Suzanne's sister died after a long illness, and she had to attend to family affairs. I also had family and business matters, including the *Dark Shadows* premiere. Our tour was fully paid for, but we managed to postpone our trip to the following October without penalty. Instead of being on the opposite side of the world on April 16, I attended my grief group session scheduled that day. Confronting the anniversary of Geoff's passing in the company of others facing similarly significant first-year occasions was fortuitous. My tearful remembrance of my husband was received with warmth and understanding; their empathy consoled me.

I went to the cemetery late that afternoon, bringing fresh flowers from the garden. Sitting on a straw mat at Geoff's grave, alone with my own thoughts, I understood I was where I needed to be on this day. While remembering the year since his death, I considered the many incremental shifts in my daily routine that reflected a life that was very changed.

I'd dropped habits and accommodations from a shared marital life that didn't suit me while living on my own. I still swam daily, but not in the late afternoon as we always had. My internal clock had adjusted to my own natural schedule, as had mealtimes and even what I chose to eat. Provisions in the cupboards no longer included oatmeal, peanut butter or boxes of pasta. I didn't linger in bed now that I was not sharing a pot of coffee and the morning newspapers. Eventually I'd moved into Geoff's office, with its view of the garden, and turned my former office into a guest room. However, I still slept on my side of the bed; the bedding on his side was smooth and untouched. The ache of missing him was still part of me, and I didn't want that to change.

I remembered that when we first started dating, Geoff had framed photographs of his wife, who had died three years earlier, propped on shelves and hanging on the walls of his house. I'd known her, too, though not well, and recalled her kindness to me years earlier on my first trip to Los Angeles only months after first meeting Geoff. In her capacity as a stringer for *Time*, she suggested I follow her in my rental car to the airport so I wouldn't get lost in rush hour traffic while picking up Ben, who was on a photographic assignment for the magazine. Afterward, she and Geoff took us out for dinner and made us feel welcome during our stay. She was magnetic, fun and caring, her beautiful, laughing face a reminder to me of a special time in my own life.

After Geoff and I began living together, I saw that he'd removed all the pictures of Barbara except those on the desk in his office. "It's not necessary to do that," I told him one evening. "This was her home. She's part of our lives and should be remembered."

I think it was the word "remembered" that hit Geoff and made him weep. "Forgetting is what you fear," he said. And as painful as memories were, I dreaded a time when I didn't feel a searing ache at missing Geoff, or couldn't recall the sound of his voice or the fragrant warmth of his skin.

With insights gained through grief group sessions and time on my own to reflect, I was easing into living as a single while still cherishing Geoff's memory as a significant force in my life. I was determined to seek out new endeavors, to adapt to life on my own, but I'd never want to erase all the poignant, intimate reminders of how we'd lived together.

Chapter Fifteen

With our departure for Beijing confirmed for September 30, *If not now, when?* became an exuberant reality crowding out thoughts about anything other than planning for our big trip. Suzanne and I filled out long passenger-information forms, secured travel insurance, booked business-class flights using miles and began reading books and trolling the Internet for travel tips on China. Throughout the summer months, we exchanged a blizzard of emails and met often for Happy Hour to go over plans for our trip. I also invited Suzanne to spend a long weekend with me in my small New York apartment to determine if we could manage to share hotel rooms on our lengthy tour; we could. *Whew.*

In an email to Suzanne, I joked about the old saying that all an actor had to do to book a job was buy a nonrefundable ticket. Suzanne, who had worked as a newscaster and an actress before going to law school, had decided after retiring from law to return to acting. I was also getting acting work, and we were both writing books. When a close friend died unexpectedly, I had to extend my stay in New York to assist in handling her estate. Each unforeseen incident was a fresh reminder that something could happen to prevent either of us from going on the trip. We agreed that if that happened we'd postpone and rebook—the answer to "if not now, when?" would just have to be "later."

A timely email from our travel agent reminded us to apply for our Chinese visas, which we did in person, spending a long morning at the Chinese consulate providing lengthy application forms with information on our flights, hotels and itinerary. The trip now felt real enough for us to give serious consideration to packing. Suzanne and I intended to travel with only carry-on luggage; however, the twenty-two pound carry-on weight limit, even for business class, and the prohibition against bringing *any* liquid in a carry-on aboard flights within China discouraged us. Our travel agent also pointed out that while traveling coach on our intra-China flights (we had five scheduled), the overheads likely wouldn't accommodate larger carry-on bags. Our intense flurry of texts and emails, much of it related to the size and weight of suitcases, only contributed to my escalating excitement—China! An hour before leaving for the airport, I changed suitcases, discarding a third of what I'd packed, and still brought too much.

Suzanne, who is far more detail minded than I am, managed to secure seats aboard a Japan Airlines flight departing Los Angeles a day earlier, giving us an extra day in Beijing to catch up on sleep before our tour officially started. We took a selfie of the two of us, grinning like schoolgirls in our roomy business-class accommodations, tucking into champagne and an array of hors d'oeuvres. A typhoon delayed us on our stopover in Tokyo; by the time our connecting flight arrived in Beijing, it was well past midnight. I was grateful that at least we'd arrived a day early. Aching with fatigue, we trailed through a vast, silent and dimly lit airport that had essentially shut down for the night, hoping our prearranged transfer to the hotel was still waiting for us. This was not a trip Geoff could have handled, even had touring China been on his list of travel adventures.

In the morning, feeling remarkably well rested and energetic, we set out to explore Beijing on our own, pocketing a handy address card from our hotel to show a taxi driver in case we got lost. Using an illustrated map and guidebook, we wandered through a tangle of backstreets locating one cultural landmark after another until midafternoon.

We'd been told that a visit to the Sanlitun Yashou Clothing Market was a "must do" in Beijing, but we couldn't find it. Suzanne stopped a middle-aged woman hurrying down the street to ask directions. The woman laughed and said, "You're standing in front of it." She was Spanish, her English excellent, and told us she served with the diplomatic corps at the nearby Spanish Embassy. We introduced ourselves, and she gave us a few shopping tips, encouraging us to bargain vigorously, before saying, "Good luck in there!"

The vast market was composed of five floors jam-packed with stalls selling clothing, leather goods, shoes and novelty items—paradise if you are a bargain shopper. We made our way to the sections Paola had recommended. The sheer magnitude of the space, with its noise and teeming crowd, was overwhelming. Two hours later we emerged with a new handbag for each of us and a silk jacket for Suzanne. Then, serendipity: we ran into Paola again on the street, this time on her way home from the embassy. After chatting a few minutes, we asked if she could recommend a good place for Chinese massage. She led us to a tranquil, beautifully designed spa nearby and then decided to have a massage herself. Afterward, she invited us to her apartment for drinks, showing us the exquisite collection of art and Chinese artifacts she'd acquired during her years stationed in Beijing. Later, over dinner at a neighborhood restaurant, Paola spoke knowledgeably about Chinese culture and current affairs while introducing us to our first genuine Chinese meal.

We lingered over dinner as Paola gave us an invaluable immersion course in the China we would experience over the coming two weeks, addressing customs, culture, environmental issues and the growing wealth gap that we would witness on our excursions into rural areas. Paola, who had traveled extensively throughout China's interior, alerted us to some of the spectacular sights we'd see on our river cruise. It was rare luck to meet her our first day in China, the sort of chance encounter Geoff had prized on our travels, valuing firsthand referrals above any guidebook. Suzanne and I stayed in touch with Paola by email after we returned home, hoping we might someday have an opportunity to show her around Los Angeles.

We'd been warned about China's air pollution and already felt its toxic effects in Beijing. Itchy eyes, a foul taste and tightness in the chest reminded us of the smog we'd experienced in Southern California before emission-control procedures began taking effect in the early 1980s. Largely due to China's reliance on coal, thick, dirty clouds of pollution would obliterate our aerial view of the country during our interior flights. As we would walk the streets of cities and villages, the intense, leaden smog brought on by ramped-up industry would act as a heavy, black curtain, obscuring shrines and sites of interest until we were almost upon them. A metaphor for China's own unwieldly reemergence from isolation, the almost-impenetrable veil reminded me to look beyond what I could readily see.

The following morning we began our official guided tour of Beijing with a walk through Tiananmen Square, a one-hundred-acre public space that can accommodate over one million people—and quite possibly did the day we were there. Our visit happened to coincide with National Day, the equivalent of the Fourth of July, commemorating October 1, 1949, when the People's Republic of China was inaugurated with a victory ceremony in Tiananmen Square. We could barely move through the jostling throngs of Chinese on holiday in Beijing's Forbidden City, an imperial palace complex of gardens, courtyards and 9,999 spectacular rooms completed in 1420. Home to China's rulers in the Ming and Qing dynasties, the palace was closed to outsiders for five centuries, protected by a wide moat and a twenty-six-foot-high wall.

The China we experienced on the first day of our grand tour could be summed up in four words: Vast. Ancient. Crowded. Exhilarating!

We traveled to Badaling the following day to visit a spectacular section of the Great Wall of China, and afterward visited the Sacred Way, a tree-lined avenue guarded by massive sculptures of elephants, lions and camels leading to the Ming dynasty tombs. Once again, we navigated through throngs of Chinese on Golden Week holiday, everyone avidly taking photographs. As often as not, Suzanne and I obligingly posed for pictures with Chinese tourists, who found two tall blondes a novelty. We would exchange smiles and awkward greetings, trying our best to say *"nǐ hǎo"* for "hello" and *"syeh-syeh"* for "thank you."

After touring Old Beijing's *hutongs* (ancient alleyways) in rickshaws, we wandered the narrow back streets of these traditional neighborhoods on our own. Three-wheeled vehicles of every description, some so fanciful they looked like handcrafted toys, whizzed around us as we took in street vendors sitting on stools cooking food in open pots or hawking silk bags, scarves and tasseled shawls. As we walked past an open door, a woman preparing a meal in her small, cramped kitchen caught my eye and beckoned us to enter. We did, nodding and smiling as we watched her form small rounds of dough into dumplings and drop them into a steaming kettle. Throughout our trip, Suzanne and I sought out these random personal interactions that provided rare glimpses into the quotidian lives of Chinese people.

We flew to Xi'an and toured the mausoleum where Emperor Qin Shi Huang was laid to rest over two thousand years ago. Suzanne and I slowly traversed the raised perimeter walkway, mesmerized by the breathtaking enormity of the necropolis where the Terra-Cotta Army had been uncovered on farmland in the 1970s. The dim half-light cast an otherworldly pall over the thousands of life-size terra-cotta cavalry, archers and infantry buried with the emperor, each man and horse molded with individual features. Often, caught up in a moment such as this, I would sense Geoff at my side, leaning against the railings with me, and feel a wave of blinding grief. How he would have delighted in seeing this glorious spectacle, his hand reaching for mine and giving it a squeeze.

In Chongqing, a mountain city and gateway to the Yangtze, we boarded our ship for a three-day cruise. We would travel one hundred and fifty miles along a scenic stretch of the river through Three Gorges, cruising first through Qutang Gorge, the shortest, narrowest and most spectacular of the three large gorges. We sailed through the night, disembarking midday for a visit to Shibaozhai Temple, an extraordinary twelve-story red pavilion built in 1650 along the Yangtze. Then we boarded a smaller boat for an excursion through the Lesser Three Gorges, accessed by sailing through Wu Gorge, an enchanting, ravishingly beautiful natural work of art.

Renowned for its magnificent scenery and limestone ridges, Wu Gorge is as mystical and surreal as scenes depicted in the Chinese silk wall hangings inspired by these lush, steep cliffs. I leaned against the railings on the top deck of the ferry and gazed up at the misty peaks of high mountains, hoping to catch a glimpse of the mysterious hanging coffins tucked into the forested slopes. Yet I was also mindful that, below the swirling river water, we were sailing over ancient dwellings, some more than four thousand years old, which had been sacrificed to the Three Gorges Dam, the world's largest hydroelectric project. Since the damming of the river, a project begun in 1994 and completed in 2012, the water has risen some 263 feet, necessitating the mass relocation of 1.3 million people from their homes in more than fifteen hundred cities, towns and villages. The controversial dam flooded archaeological and cultural sites, causing significant ecological disruption and an increased risk of landslides.

All of our tour guides were knowledgeable and well-spoken, several of them far more candid than I had expected when addressing questions concerning political, social, ecological and cultural issues. Our guide on this portion of the tour volunteered that we were sailing over his birthplace, that his grandmother and parents had been relocated a great distance from their lifelong home. His voice betrayed ongoing grief over the loss of their home and separation from family and community. I gazed back up at the majestic mountains, musing on the significance of a single human lifetime in a country with a three-thousand-year written history, that is home to more than 1.3 billion people, then parsed that to grieve over my own loss. Life is fleeting and the world moves on.

Midafternoon, we boarded a flat-bottomed boat for a cruise through a narrow gorge. With a quick nod of his head, the pilot permitted me to pass through a narrow doorway to the front deck of the boat, where I could sit by myself and have an unobstructed view. I perched on a fuel canister, my feet propped against a low ridge, enjoying the solitude and close-up view of river life gliding by. Midway through our whirlwind tour of China, I cherished lulls when I could simply soak up the moment, taking in the sharp tang of the gray-green river water and the moist crispness of the air. The sensory overload of crowded streets and cacophony of unfamiliar sounds, smells and tastes made these quiet respites welcome. I focused on individual people walking along the covered footpaths clinging to the edges of the cliffs and was caught up in brief glimpses of monkeys and goats visible through the mists on the bluffs. I watched figures along the shore at work washing clothes in the river water. I exchanged nods and a wave of greeting with a man and woman sailing past in their shallow boat, and hoped I could preserve such particular moments of connection to carry home with me.

I also thought of Geoff and imagined him sitting next to me, the two of us pointing out sights we wanted to share. Some people on board were dealing with health issues, but I would have considered this trip too arduous for travel with a wheelchair. While the hotels we stayed in were all five star plus, with all the amenities one could desire, the pace of the tour itself would have been too grueling for Geoff. I shuddered at the thought of dealing with a fall or other medical emergency on this trip, let alone the anxiety of handling any "new normal" that cropped up.

Then I reminded myself that we'd managed trips to Russia, Italy, Paris, Prague and London, among many other destinations, and handily dealt with problems that arose. Even with all the hazards inherent in our last big trip together to South America, we'd coped very well. It occurred to me that the chief difference was my changed perspective. I was now viewing our far-flung travels in hindsight, wondering how in the world we'd done it! But then I had to admit that if Geoff had felt a burning desire to visit China, we'd probably have met the challenges and made it work.

That evening, Suzanne and I stood on deck in a misty drizzle, not wanting to miss a thing as we sailed through the five-stage locks of the Three Gorges Dam. The following day I gave my new hip a workout on a long trek surveying the mammoth engineering masterpiece. I also climbed winding ancient stairs to the top of a pagoda, trekked through a mountaintop village and strolled along scenic pathways that offered breathtaking panoramas of the countryside.

I embraced every opportunity to mingle with Chinese people. In Jingzhou, I welcomed the chance to visit an elementary school. I joined children in their classrooms, sharing a desk with one young girl who shyly asked to try on my sun hat, and participated in their games on the playground—a joyful experience. At other times during our trip, Suzanne and I attended theatre, opera and dance performances with largely Chinese audiences. And in Wuhan, our last stop before flying to Shanghai, we joined throngs of local visitors at the Hubei Provincial Museum to hear the music of ancient bronze bells.

In Shanghai, China's largest city and one of the world's most important ports, we stayed in The Westin Bund Center, another luxurious five-star hotel with a dazzling buffet. We spent a morning touring the Old City of Shanghai and visited the Shanghai Museum, viewing ancient bronzes, ceramics, calligraphy, paintings and a jade gallery. In the afternoon, we went to the magnificent Yuyuan Garden, five acres of winding paths and intricately carved pavilions, which dates back to the Ming dynasty.

But after our lengthy guided tour, Suzanne and I wanted to set out to explore on our own. On our walk through a park, we ran into two delightful, very pretty Chinese students, who asked if we'd pose for selfies with them. The young women said they'd both applied to complete their studies at an American university—would we permit them to walk with us so they could practice their language skills? We readily agreed, embracing another opportunity to spend time with local Chinese.

One of the girls excitedly told us how fortunate we were to be visiting Shanghai during the Tea Festival, a very special tradition that few foreign visitors had an opportunity to experience. She remembered that the best place to partake in a traditional tea ceremony happened to be nearby. What luck!

Off we went with our new best friends, darting through twisting side streets until we arrived at a shabby building with a narrow entranceway down a short flight of steps. The tiny room we were ushered into was dark and airless, pungent with the dank aroma of steeped tea. Four bamboo chairs were set in front of a narrow countertop facing a wall of flimsy shelving holding tea canisters and petite black pots and cups.

The women anticipated our wariness about the close quarters, whispering that fancy-looking teahouses were for tourists, but this establishment was celebrated for observing traditional customs. They showed great deference toward an inscrutable elderly woman behind the counter, who seemed none too pleased to see us, explaining that she spoke no English and wasn't accustomed to serving Westerners. We took it that our presence was tolerated only because of our sweet young friends. The door was shut and we were handed menus, which were, of course, in Chinese. The girls insisted we partake of the "Festival Special" and sample everything, but by then the stifling room and their increasingly controlling behavior made us both uneasy. Feeling trapped, I looked around, sensing someone watching us—then spotted men's shoes on the floor behind a curtained archway.

In full-blown panic, I bolted out of my chair. "Suzanne, we're late! We have to get back! They're expecting us!"

Suzanne was on her feet in an instant. We attempted to make our scramble for the door decorous and polite. "So sorry! Really, we can't stay. How much?" Suzanne pressed Chinese currency on the counter, and we were off, still apologizing profusely as we hurried up the steps. We couldn't walk fast enough—except we had no idea where we were going.

Several streets away, panting and out of breath, we slowed down. "So sorry, Suzanne, but I had to get out of there. Someone was watching us from behind that curtain. All I could think is that we were going to be drugged and dragged off into captivity!"

"Shanghaied?" Suzanne laughed. "White slavery? Who would want us? Robbed, maybe . . ."

"Those girls were so nice. I hope they're okay."

"But imagine what the old lady is saying about us," Suzanne said. "Not our finest moment."

It occurred to us that the girls may have been conning us into paying for a costly tea ceremony, but we were more concerned about the poor impression we'd made as untrusting, ill-mannered Americans. Suzanne wished she'd left more money than the equivalent of five dollars, but we both agreed the experience had been creepy, no matter how authentic the tea ceremony.

That evening, while attending a performance by the famed Shanghai Acrobatic Troupe, we sheepishly confided our misadventure to Dan and Scott, two shipboard friends. "It's a scam!" Dan said, astonished at our gullibility. "Didn't you read the warnings about being inveigled into these tea ceremonies? You were lucky to get out of there for five bucks."

After the performance, the four of us strolled along the Bund, a glittery waterfront thoroughfare lit against the night sky, taking in the shimmering array of architectural styles that spanned Gothic and baroque to beaux arts and art deco. I was intent on visiting the Fairmont Peace Hotel, formerly the Cathay Hotel—the most prestigious hotel in Shanghai before 1949, and where Sir Noël Coward wrote *Private Lives*. The newly refurbished hotel was a glorious masterpiece of art deco design, the style in which Geoff and I had decorated our New York apartment. I could almost feel his hand on my shoulder, guiding me through the breathtakingly beautiful lobby.

Geoff, who loved martinis and traditional jazz, would have felt at home in the hotel's Jazz Bar, a retro boîte with a wood-beamed ceiling, long bar and mahogany furnishings. I could envision Humphrey Bogart in a white dinner jacket telling Dooley Wilson to "play it, Sam." Geoff's favorite bar bet, which frequently won him a martini on the house, was to correctly identify the pianist—Elliot Carpenter—who actually played "As Time Goes By" in *Casablanca*. Odds-on, the veteran bartender mixing our cocktails would not have been stumped. The six-piece band, composed of elderly Chinese musicians (average age mid-eighties) clad in vintage tuxes, played traditional '20s and '30s jazz numbers that had Dan and I on our feet dancing.

It was late by the time we left the Jazz Bar, but instead of walking the most direct route to our hotel, the four of us zigzagged through the dark back streets, me in the lead with no idea where we were. Lost, with no map in hand, I turned another corner and came across a sandwich board printed in English with the words "Happy Hour." It stopped me in my tracks.

I saw that I was standing in front of a bar called the House of Blues and Jazz. Without waiting for the others, I bounded up the stairs of the two-story brick building to look inside. The dark wood interior had a massive carved staircase and was hung with vintage posters and Jazz Age ephemera—my kind of place! My friends, exhausted after a full day of sightseeing, indulged my plea to have a nightcap and hear some music. The place was jammed, but we climbed the stairs to a second-floor gallery with stained-glass windows that overlooked the bandstand and crowded dance floor. A band playing traditional jazz struck up "Stardust," and I was awash in memories of Artie Shaw—and Geoff. How I wished he were with me—and then I knew he was.

I looked around, sure that somewhere in the crush of people lining the bar I'd find him wearing his safari jacket and black Italian cap, a martini straight-up in hand, thrilling to the music. Would he spot me, as he always had when I joined him at Birdland, and make room for me next to him at the bar?

I stood transfixed in that Shanghai bar, the vibrant music of the swing band embracing me, flushing my cheeks with memories of Geoff with his arm around my shoulders, his fingers rhythmically squeezing my hand. Of course, this is where he'd be. I'd found him and, for a few moments, we were together again.

We flew from Shanghai to the picturesque city of Guilin, which literally means "Forest of Sweet Osmanthus," named for the small, fragrant evergreen tree. We stayed at the luxurious five-star Shangri-La Hotel, our suite of rooms rivaling the size of my New York apartment. Dinner was a multicourse meal from a vast choice of buffet stations featuring Chinese and international cuisine. The following day, leaving the lavish hotel setting made me even more aware of the huge wealth gap that was so evident on our excursion into the countryside.

We cruised the Li River, glimpsing idyllic scenes of rural Chinese life, where farmers tended water buffalo and women washed clothes along the shores. The forested, limestone hills were breathtaking, and the ever-present haze cast a mystical aura over the dramatic landscape. But up close, walking the dusty streets of a small village choked with souvenir vendors, I was again struck by the extreme poverty and deprivation.

Our last few days were spent in Hong Kong, staying at the Kowloon Shangri-La hotel in a room with a mesmerizing harbor view of boats and dazzling skyline. We visited the waterfront township of Aberdeen and boarded a sampan for a tour of the "floating village" with its colorful junks, fishing boats, lavish yachts and traditional flat-bottomed sampans. My Korean friend, Christine, who lives in Hong Kong with her British husband and two children, spent an entire day showing us her favorite places. She took us to the enormous blocks-long Ladies Market in Kowloon, where Suzanne and I indulged ourselves buying novelty gifts. We also visited Christine's home, joined her for dinner at a local restaurant, and saw Hong Kong from a local's perspective.

The following afternoon, we departed on a Cathay Pacific flight, our luggage bulging, my iPad loaded with journal notes and hundreds of photos of our amazing trip. Home again, groggy, jet-lagged and too wired to sleep, I sent an email to Suzanne:

Hey, still speaking . . . still friends . . . what a fantastic time! Can't believe we were in Hong Kong yesterday. Showered off the last of China and stepped on a scale . . . wow! I weigh less than when I left. Does this mean bowls of noodles, rice and three croissants a day (yes, the Shangri-La turns out a great croissant!) is the secret? . . . where to next, my friend?

Suddenly wide awake in the early hours of the morning, it struck me that the last bed I'd slept in was half a world away in Hong Kong and had come with a harbor view—and croissants. The memory of those lavish hotel breakfast buffets made me smile, even as I glanced at a framed picture of Geoff on the bedside table. It had been just over eighteen months since he'd passed away, and I'd taken my first big trip without him. As the thought sank in, I expected to feel a thud of grief and terrible longing. Instead, I gazed at his sunny face and felt a wave of love. "Wish you were here," I whispered, swinging my legs out of bed. "I miss you."

Fortified with coffee and bundled up against the autumn chill, I gathered flowers from the garden and headed to the cemetery, arriving just as the guard unlocked the entry gates. As a rule, tears would sting my eyes and I'd weep even before parking my car, but not on this morning. The realization hit me as I walked across the wet grass and dropped my mat next to Geoff's grave. Instead of aching sorrow, I felt a rush of emotion akin to what I experienced whenever I hadn't seen him for a while—an hour, an afternoon—and he came back into my life again. I plopped down on the straw mat and began arranging the flowers I'd brought.

"Guess where I've been?" I smiled, my eyes brimming at the memory of the Shanghai jazz bar. "But then, you were there, too."

PART THREE

THIS IS LIFE, NOT A DRESS REHEARSAL.

Chapter Sixteen

I often joke that when my phone rings, I answer, "Yes! Where? I'm on my way." It's an actor's typical reply when an agent calls, but these days I make every effort to respond to daily life like that.

My memories of Geoff are still sharp. I recall the sound of his voice and the look in his eyes, and see him as the funny, strong, vibrant love of my life, just as I hoped I could one day remember him. The grieving that began in the caregiving years and the awful sorrow after he died aren't forgotten, either, but with time, those painful memories have woven themselves into the fabric of my everyday life. I carry it all with me, melding everything from the past with all that's happening as I move on with life.

"If not now, when?" is a motto I've come to live by, informing most of the decisions I make these days. Why put something off? What am I saving up for? Essentially I'm quoting my friend Allan, a widower I met in my grief group, who still joins me for Happy Hour long after we both stopped attending our Monday sessions. (No, he's not the same fellow who asked me out!)

For Allan, "if not now, when?" has been a guiding principle throughout his life. Sixty-two years to the day after he left high school a month early to enlist in the navy during World War II, he returned to his old Los Angeles neighborhood to join the graduating class of 2006. He regaled me with stories: "One of the senior girls at the graduation rehearsal said to me, 'My date and I would be honored if you would go to the prom with us. We have a limo.' I thanked her, but said it would be past my bedtime," he said with a laugh.

Though I'd never met his wife, Alice, I felt I got to know her quite well through his stories about their life together. He described how, early in their marriage, he'd put a sign in the window closing the business for two weeks to go traveling: "And guess what? The world didn't come to an end."

The two loved adventure travel and went everywhere, immersing themselves in the local culture and striving to blend in. On canal boats in Europe, they'd operate the locks on their own, tie up at the riverside and then bike into a village for dinner or to pick up milk and wine. If they opened the door of a restaurant in a foreign country and heard English spoken, they didn't go in.

They hiked in the Himalayas, and Alice, who was a marathon runner, would lead the way, hopping from one slippery rock to the next when crossing a river. The first indication that Alice was ill came during a trip to the Galápagos Islands when she seemed unsteady and fell a few times, which was unlike her. Even that didn't stop them: when they could no longer enjoy the challenges of adventure trips, they took cruises. Their last was through the Panama Canal from Fort Lauderdale back to Los Angeles.

Now a hardy ninety years old, Allan is an inspiration to me. He and I still get together for Happy Hour on days after he and his service dog, GG, have volunteered at the veterans hospital. But often the two are traveling, usually to Hawaii for weeks at a time. His overriding motto is "You can't hold out for 'someday,' because it may never come," and it's this sage advice that spurs me on.

In truth, my telephone doesn't ring as much as it once did, leaving aside the fact that texting and email have become more popular modes of communication. The reality is that my life is no longer as socially active as it was when I was part of a couple. Newly widowed, I wasn't necessarily up to attending dinner parties, arriving and leaving on my own, with constant reminders of Geoff's absence. My emotions were too fragile to handle bright dinner-party conversation.

One evening, I joined two couples for dinner in a restaurant. As we sat down at the table, one of the men looked around, genuinely bewildered, and asked, "How come we're only five tonight?"

"Because Geoff couldn't make it," I said.

We all laughed, unselfconsciously as close friends can. The man covered my hand with his and said, "Oh, of course. I knew something wasn't right."

In that tender moment I almost lost it, but if I had, it would have been okay. These were among our dearest friends, and they felt Geoff's loss, too. But with those who have always known you as part of a couple, a missing partner is like an absent band member, the bass note absent, or an ingredient left out of a cake, its flavor now off. I instinctively tried to fill in for Geoff, to be two and make up the difference, but that doesn't work, either.

As self-reliant as I imagine myself to be, finding my comfort level as a newly single person did not come easily. It was inevitable that customary dinner invitations with couples soon morphed into lunches, seldom with both halves of a twosome present. A woman would meet me for dinner only when her spouse was working late or out of town; otherwise it was lunch. Dinner-party invitations grew sparse. I thought hard about whether I had, even subconsciously, excluded singles from my own gatherings, but I was relieved to recall many occasions when I'd seated three, five or seven guests at my table. Some friends, I knew, felt awkward having an extra woman at the table, which somehow isn't the same as having an extra man at the table.

Do men have it easier? As a fresh widower, Geoff claimed he'd never wined or dined so well, his dance card always full. He'd appreciated the flood of invitations for the diversion they provided; he had only to mark his calendar and show up. However, when we began dating three years after Barbara died, a glance in his freezer stocked with Stouffer's ready-made dinners told a different story. By then the shine had worn off being in demand as everyone's spare man and the expectations that often came with a hostess's attempts at matchmaking. He got tired of being fixed up and preferred eating at home alone.

Over Happy Hour one afternoon, Allan and I discussed how to handle the pitfalls of singlehood social life, which we agreed is as fraught as it was when we were callow teenagers. Allan confided that after Alice died, a parade of his wife's bridge-club set arrived at his door with casseroles. The food was a calling card, and reciprocating with a dinner out was construed as an overture to romance and couple-hood.

I recounted a humorous experience when a girlfriend called to complain to me that my former husband, Ben, had not followed up with a woman she'd matched him with at a dinner party. "She's very interested in him, and he said he'd call her, but hasn't!" I promised I'd look into it. It was testament to our cordial relationship, despite being divorced for decades, that I called him to explain spare-man-dinner-guest etiquette: "If you said you'd call her, you have to call her, but come up with a nice excuse for not seeing her," I told him. "Don't keep her dangling!"

We shared a good laugh, but all I could think was that I didn't want to be on either end of such a call. I had no interest in dating or being fixed up.

Chapter Seventeen

Happy Hour had eased me back out into the world, but I missed cooking and entertaining at home, which had been such a significant part of my social life with Geoff. I began inviting pals for casual meals in the kitchen and in the garden around the outdoor grill. These early evening get-togethers evolved into what we dubbed the Monday Night Supper Club, a communal gathering involving about seven of us, who all loved to cook and enjoyed good food and wine. David, a chef, generally coordinated the menu, but we all pitched in, supplying the ingredients and rolling up our sleeves to prepare the meal—a recipe for chaos in the kitchen, but great fun.

Aside from David and Tim, who had married in our garden some years earlier, we were all singles and old friends who relished a chance to show off our signature dishes. *Seasonal* and *organic* were key words, all of us delighting in bringing to the table something enticing we'd found at a farmers market or artisanal shop. Group cleanup and shared leftovers were part of the bargain.

It was a joy to see the house and garden come alive again with laughter and good times. Friends made a point of wearing some article of clothing that had once belonged to Geoff, and we'd occasionally raise a glass to toast him. He still felt very present in our lives.

"We live in a 'couples world,'" my friend Roz told me. "The price you pay for the joy of being with someone you love is the terrible pain that comes when it ends." After her husband died of cancer, she felt like an amputee, missing a part of herself without Bill. "I sobbed . . . couldn't cease sobbing for some three years."

The turning point for Roz came when she contracted pneumonia. On her own and very ill, she tried to drive herself to the hospital but passed out on the way. Her car grazed a tree, and a passerby called medics. The accident made for a sort of intervention, a jolt that liberated her from the terrible crying. She looked around their house on Martha's Vineyard and realized that although she and Bill would never again sit on the porch together with a glass of wine, she didn't want anyone else living in Bill's house. Her solution was a change of scene, finding a new place to live where she could start fresh.

After a lengthy period of tears and grief, I reached my own turning point, but it didn't happen as dramatically for me as it had for Roz. My light-bulb moment occurred quite literally when I flipped a switch and a lamp illuminated a storage area in my house that I seldom entered, and for good reason. A sort of "Fibber McGee's closet," it was crammed with things that weren't mine and that I didn't use. I had somehow become the keeper of other people's stuff, items that had belonged to Geoff's deceased parents, his brother, Barbara and her parents and children, and even Ben and various other friends and family members. All of it had been left in our house for safekeeping, but it was unlikely anyone had ever intended to reclaim the goods.

The contraband included generations of old tennis rackets, school trophies, scrapbooks, ski boots and snorkeling gear, pennants and posters, outmoded electronic paraphernalia, knickknacks of every description and a slide projector with trays of transparencies of people I didn't know and places I'd never been. I'm not a hoarder, nor can I abide clutter, but the reason I had not thrown any of these things away was because they didn't belong to me. I had cupboards full of other people's wedding gifts, with monogrammed initials on linens and silver that weren't mine, and china patterns I would never have chosen and would never use.

Lest I throw stones at glass houses, I should admit I also discovered a keepsake trove of my own. My mother, in one of her own "clear out the attic" phases, had shipped a box to me that contained my junior and senior prom corsages, a rose bouquet from my senior high school class play, church-confirmation corsage and Spring Fling sophomore nosegay. I had preserved them all using various methods (wax, borax, air drying, glycerin) as a science experiment in my senior year, and I couldn't bear to throw my collection away.

It was time to declutter and make my living space my own. I set aside items I thought Barbara's children would want and disposed of the rest (except for my floral science experiment) one way or another. Clearing out took time, but eventually cupboards and shelves were bare and I had some empty closets and drawers. It was liberating, and set wheels of thought in motion. I loved our house and had no intention of selling, but there was no reason to be tied down by it. I could lease it for a while and start afresh somewhere. Or travel.

But there were also still adventures to be had close to home. My literary agent encouraged me to launch a mystery series based on a novel, *Down and Out in Beverly Heels,* I'd begun about a self-made woman who has everything, loses everything and ends up living on the streets of Beverly Hills in her "Ritz-Volvo." The idea sprang from volunteer work I was doing with the homeless program in my church. I put my homeless and destitute lead character in further jeopardy by having the FBI investigate her possible criminal involvement in the very scam that had cost her everything.

Among the reasons I enjoy my work as both an actress and writer is the research involved in creating a character and bringing a story to life. I knew nothing about the FBI, but after a bit of investigation on my own, I discovered an online application for the FBI Citizens Academy and enrolled. I was accepted into the program and, over the course of fascinating weekly sessions, absorbed all I could from the special agents instructing us in everything from firearms training on a shooting range to procedural methods used in investigating crime. I took a lie-detector test, experienced simulated shooting scenarios and fired weapons I hope never to come across again in real life—but I'm now familiar enough with their heft, operation, "kick" and killing capabilities to write about them. I also drew on my observations and personal chats with individual FBI agents for perspective and insight I could use in developing characters in my story.

Another dividend of that extraordinary training was meeting and working with some fifty FBI agents and twenty-two other classmates, all terrific people with every sort of background and knowledge. My initial intent may have been to research a book, but I found real value in personally engaging with people I would never otherwise meet and exposing myself to stimulating new relationships and experiences.

Gretchen Urnes Beito, a writer several years my senior and a widow whose husband died three years before Geoff, echoed some of my sentiments over a long lunch during a visit to Los Angeles. "Writing saved me," she revealed. Throughout the many years she was a caregiver for Gene, who had Parkinson's disease, she wrote a column, Prairie Rambling, for the *Thief River Falls Times*, her hometown Minnesota newspaper. In the years since her husband's death, she's written children's books about handmade dolls and various articles and books on local history subjects.

I'd worked closely with Gretchen many years earlier while editing and publishing *Coya Come Home*, her biography of Coya Knutson, Minnesota's first congresswoman and our mutual childhood hero. Over lunch during her visit, we discussed the newly revised paperback edition, with a foreword by Walter F. Mondale, that would be published that summer. But much of our conversation centered on how we were going about finding new direction in our lives now that we were on our own.

For Gretchen, that meant not only nurturing ties with her three children and many grandchildren, but time spent on her own pursuits— largely writing and traveling. On the first anniversary of Gene's death, Gretchen was on a Road Scholar tour of Australia. She remained close to friends in Northern Minnesota, enjoying her garden and long walks, but she'd made new friends during winter months spent in Arizona. She continued to book tours to faraway places, appreciating the opportunity to travel with people as open to new cultural experiences as she was.

In the wake of long chats with Gretchen, I began to consider other options open to me. My daily life centered on writing, which I enjoyed, but the long hours at my desk had become routine and isolating. I was finding it very easy to stay home, spending time in my garden or reading for diversion and experiencing a little too much comfort in solitude. I was becoming reclusive, which isn't healthy. I still traveled occasionally, but aside from my trip to China with Suzanne, most often I was revisiting places familiar to me. What was holding me back from exploring new destinations? While I'm comfortable traveling on my own, I recognized that much of my pleasure comes from sharing the experience with someone else. Perhaps joining tour groups was the answer.

But, like both Roz and Gretchen, I was beginning to think a lengthier change of scene was in order.

I was lucky that I already had a ready-made change of scene waiting for me in New York. Our apartment, essentially the size of a well-appointed junior hotel suite, had suited our needs perfectly on Geoff's frequent business trips to New York when he was publishing the magazine. Later, fitted with handicap aids and equipment, it provided us with a safe, comfortable refuge in a city Geoff loved to visit.

On my next trip to New York, I took a closer look at the apartment and my neighborhood, gauging the appeal of making my home in the city. Oddly enough, we'd always treated the apartment much like a weekend retreat, leaving little behind after our relatively brief stays. Closets and drawers were essentially empty, kitchen cupboards stocked with little more than the basics. Somehow that made the move even more enticing. Instead of having to clear out stuff, I would be making our apartment a homier place for a longer-term stay.

The move was appealing for practical financial considerations, too. It wasn't lost on me that, newly widowed, I'd created a fictional character who was my alter ego—the valiant, resourceful, unvanquished woman I hoped I could be if I were to somehow lose my home and everything I'd worked so hard to achieve. Plumbing my own worst fears, I empathized with the gritty underbelly of despair a homeless woman would face living in her car undetected, the roof over her head coming with four wheels and a dashboard but none of the amenities necessary to cope with daily life. Through my volunteer work, I'd witnessed women who were "homeless and hiding it" eking out a day-to-day existence in affluent neighborhoods where they'd once resided in safety and comfort.

I was vividly aware of how little it takes to lose everything: widowhood, divorce, catastrophic illness or accident, bad investments, career meltdown, natural disaster, or a combination of these could spell calamity.

When the book was published almost exactly two years after Geoff's death, I was gratified that in my own book club and at book signings, discussions invariably turned to the issues of coping with and surviving loss. The talks I gave at various events became an extension of the sorts of conversations I'd had about these matters with caregivers I met in support groups and friends who were dealing with the same post-caregiving issues and concerns I was. Writing the book was personally cathartic for me and had a considerable impact on how I reevaluated my daily life and made some major changes.

I was very grateful that we'd had the financial means to provide Geoff with the medical and home care he'd required, but even with our insurance, the expenses had mounted. At the same time, my role as caregiver had meant pulling back from professional work. We'd managed well, but the combination of the increasing medical expenses and my steady loss of income had been emotionally unsettling. Despite reassurances from our accountant, I still felt insecure and uncertain. Although I was working again, I was also supporting our former lifestyle while living on my own.

I was reminded of the conversation I'd had with my mother shortly before she died, the one leading to her admission that some of her most satisfying, enjoyable years had been after my father passed away. Living on her own, she'd been cautious at first, taking it a step at a time until she felt secure about budgeting money for hair appointments, dinners out and travel. She'd never spent frivolously, but after a while, she found she could indulge herself with the better brand of hand lotion, afford nice shoes and dine out occasionally. In time, she gained confidence in her ability to support herself and handle her own affairs. It pleased her to no end to reach for the lunch check when it suited her, because she knew to the penny what she could afford.

I was clearly my mother's daughter, cautious at first but gaining confidence as time went on. Still, despite having a good business sense, I frequently wished I could turn to Geoff for advice on financial matters. Eventually, for my own peace of mind, I set about altering my lifestyle.

A real estate broker helped me see the home I'd lived in for more than twenty-five years through the eyes of a potential renter. Once I depersonalized my house and made a few minor repairs, the broker found suitable tenants, and I enthusiastically packed up for my move. New York would be both a place I'd shared with Geoff and an intriguing new adventure. I couldn't help but think he'd applaud me for embarking on this bold next chapter in my life.

Chapter Eighteen

Wait, what just happened? Why was I so happy? In New York I did not miss palm trees or driving a car. I loved walking everywhere and occasionally riding a bus or the subway. I felt liberated living in a more confined space, free of all the chores involved in managing a house. I still spent long days writing, but taking a break meant walking down the street to buy an apple or banana off a barrow or a strolling by the river. I was back living full-time in my old neighborhood, where almost fifty years earlier I'd filmed a Coca-Cola commercial in the florist shop on the corner. Everything was both new and familiar at the same time, and I didn't have a return airline ticket to remind me this wasn't my real home.

On impulse, I called an acting teacher I'd studied with in New York. I reminded him that I'd been in his class only two months before being cast in *Dark Shadows*. I'd had to drop out because of the demands of recording a live television show, but I had always regretted not training with him longer. He laughed and invited me back to class: "All is forgiven!"

How great to be doing scene work with young actors just starting out and other veterans who had also returned to study with this revered teacher. At age ninety-three, he was a recent widower who still had the stamina and creative drive to teach five classes a week, an inspiration in itself.

I got to know my neighbors and made new friends. I also reunited with people I'd stayed close to over the years but had seen only sporadically on visits to New York. Among the friendships I most treasured were those with former Bunnies I'd worked with in the early days of the New York Playboy Club while I was a student. The women had formed a close-knit sisterhood over the years, one I had gratefully tapped into even from a distance. While in Los Angeles two years earlier, I had received a call from police in New York alerting me that a very close friend, who had been ill for some time, had passed away in her apartment. One immediate concern was caring for her beloved dog, elderly and distressed, that I could hear barking in the background. I made a single call to a longtime Bunny friend that was quickly transmitted through the sisterhood. Only minutes later I got a return call from one of the women offering to pick up and care for my deceased friend's dog.

I was delighted to have this vibrant, diverse, supportive group of old friends embrace my return to New York and welcome me back into their circle. I loved being invited to join these women for boisterous, fun-filled dinner parties in the garden apartment of one of the former Bunnies, a bridal milliner with a penchant for cooking elaborate, multicourse Italian feasts.

My neighbors Pamela and Diane, both single women, showed me how to make the most of all New York can offer. Pamela, an avid theatre maven, would alert me to must-see plays in out-of-the-way venues I'd otherwise miss and ask if I wanted her to pick up an extra ticket for me. Diane was quick to advise me on neighborhood events and point out good restaurants. They'd both known Geoff and were a link to the life I missed having with him, but they also helped me navigate the transition to living in a world without him.

❖   ❖   ❖

Then, something very unexpected happened. One afternoon I met a man in a hallway. I'd arrived early at a concert studio, as I invariably do. He had arrived even earlier and told me the entrance doors weren't open yet. We chatted amiably for a couple minutes without introducing ourselves. When the doors were opened, we both entered and took seats on opposite sides of the room. Afterward, we met up again riding down in the elevator. By the time we reached the ground floor, he'd invited me for a drink, and I'd said yes.

It was a blustery March evening, and he took my elbow to steer me through the crowded, windy street to a cozy bar in a French bistro. I noticed he was very tall, wore a nice suit and had blue eyes. Over glasses of good Bordeaux I learned he was an American businessman who had spent many years working in Europe and was relatively new to living in New York. I told him I'd recently moved to New York, too, but was also very familiar with the cities where he'd lived in Europe. We talked easily, sharing stories, and discovered we had a fair number of common interests. We were seemingly about the same age; his hair was salt-and-pepper, as was mine.

After more conversation and a second glass of wine, we stepped out of the restaurant into a cold drizzle. When he put me in a cab, I liked the feel of his hand on my back. Had I just been picked up? Grinning in the taxi on the way home, I realized I'd encountered a complete stranger I hoped to see again.

We'd exchanged email addresses, and we arranged to meet that weekend at a movie theatre in Tribeca to see a vintage French film. I was a bit early, but he was already there, tickets in hand. He waved to me as I crossed the street, and I hurried to meet him. I discovered he was fluent in French; I made do with subtitles. We had coffee afterward, then parted on a corner, going our separate ways. I started off in the wrong direction trying to find the subway and had to backtrack. I caught sight of him across the street, moving swiftly, hands in his pockets, his body thrust forward in the chill wind. He didn't see me, and I watched him walk away, gauging my reaction to suddenly coming across him again, no longer just a passerby on the street. A little flutter in my belly provided the answer.

We met for Sunday brunch at the same place we'd had coffee, then went for a long walk. He was easygoing, funny and enjoyed walking at a fast clip as much as I did. I was charmed and found him very attractive, but by then I'd determined he was younger than me. I hadn't divulged my age, nor had he, but as far as I could tell, he was my kid brother's age. What was I thinking? *Ridiculous!*

While I'm not particularly secretive about my age, I did feel self-conscious about the *difference* in our ages. Surely my absurd crush on this stranger would end in tears if I didn't put a stop to it at once.

But I didn't. The bossy, scrappy, reckless side of me said, *So what?* Tears, should they come, are not new to me. I function in careers that are rife with personal rejection, and I'm still standing. I'm at an age when I've weathered far worse than the horrified reaction of a would-be lover saying, "You're *how* old?" This would not kill me. If I was game for amorous adventure, I'd been presented with a prospect I couldn't ignore. After all, my head, heart and nether regions were informing me that I was smitten. I hadn't been looking for romance, but clearly I was open to it. With a *stranger* I'd met in a *hallway*.

He took me for dinner at an Italian restaurant (he spoke fluent Italian, I discovered), and catching a glimpse of the two of us in a mirrored panel, I noted that I did not look like his mother or even his older sister. How wrong could this go? He mentioned he'd been married and was divorced. He seemed interested in me, but was it romantic? Were we dating? It felt like we might be, but how would I know? It had been more than twenty-five years since I last dated.

Over the course of a couple weeks, we met for lunches, dinners and long walks, slowly getting to know each other. I took pleasure in the company of a man who was delightful, accomplished, well-educated and liked traditional jazz. One evening I introduced him to Birdland, the New York jazz haunt Geoff had favored. I arrived early to make sure we'd get a good table. I nodded to James, the bartender, and chatted with the manager, who informed me that the legendary record-producer George Avakian would be arriving to celebrate his ninety-fifth birthday. The atmosphere was festive, the place packed, and the music wonderful. An old musician friend who'd been close to Geoff joined our table, giving me a sly wink when he saw the two of us holding hands.

Later we stopped in a pub for an Irish coffee then strolled up the street, holding hands. The night air was chilly, the sky star-filled as we headed across town. Somewhere near Fifth Avenue, he pulled me close and kissed me. Any doubts or reservations I may have had vanished into woozy delirium as we kissed again. The only problem in that magical moment was that my bag was packed and I would be off to London the following day.

I felt like a lovestruck schoolgirl and didn't hide it. One day over lunch with a girlfriend at P.J. Clarke's, I confided that I'd met someone, but then faltered when trying to describe him. I realized I didn't really know him that well and had made him sound more like a travel brochure than a person. I could rattle off facts (he had business and law degrees, spoke several languages fluently and had a deep knowledge of literature, for example), but what about *him*? We hadn't met through friends. There were no personal references. We knew each other only through whatever we'd chosen to share about our backgrounds, work, family and experiences.

I started to really get to know him through email exchanges and long Skype conversations while I was in London. Distance helped. It was somehow easier to ask questions, to listen more closely to his responses and to learn about the person I was finding so very attractive. I bought him a fine woolen scarf as a gift and selected several cheeses at Neal's Yard in Covent Garden that I knew he'd like. He, in turn, offered to cook dinner for me the evening I returned to New York. I couldn't wait to see him.

On my flight home I thumbed through photos of Geoff on my iPhone. He was very much on my mind because that day happened to mark the fourth anniversary of his death. Then, shortly before we landed, I discovered I'd lost the watch Geoff had given me soon after we married. I was distraught. I knew I'd had it on when I boarded. Luckily, just before deplaning, I found the watch on the floor under my seat, its silver link strap broken. Arriving home, I went straight to the jeweler in my neighborhood, who repaired the watch strap in a matter of minutes. Later I unpacked, showered and put my watch back on, but a different link broke, and it fell off my wrist. I raced back to the jeweler.

While I waited for him to repair the watch again, it struck me that perhaps Geoff was sending me a message. I smiled at the thought he might be warning me to behave myself. Knowing Geoff, it was more likely he was telling me it was time to make the break, to move on, as he had done when he met me. In the four years since he'd passed away, I'd been getting on with life on my own, but I still felt significantly attached to Geoff and couldn't—or hadn't yet been able to—let go and truly consider having a relationship with someone else. I put my watch back on and went home.

It shouldn't have come as a surprise to me that the man I'd missed so much while in London would be a wonderful cook. He arrived at my apartment with vintage champagne and a pedigreed chicken, which he roasted with vegetables to savory perfection. I supplied the cheeses and candlelight. Dinner was delicious, and so was the night we spent together. The thought of intimacy had been horrifying, though desired; the reality was timely and transforming. I was grateful for the space of time we'd had apart and the magic of Skype that had drawn us closer.

My watchstrap stayed fixed, and I took it as a good sign.

One of my prime motivations for moving to New York was a yearning to travel more. In addition to my long-planned visit to London, I'd scheduled three more trips for that spring, each one close on the heels of the last. Every trip was significant and purposeful in its own way, but now that someone meaningful had entered my life, all the travel struck me as excessive. The melting euphoria of a new relationship was exciting enough; I was giddy at the very thought of having a boyfriend.

Only a week after returning from London, I was booked on an early-morning train to participate in an FBI field trip to Washington, DC, with a four-day tour of the FBI Academy at Quantico and CIA headquarters in Langley. I was eager to spend time with my former FBI Citizens Academy classmates and thrilled to have such rare access to Bureau headquarters. I arrived at Penn Station early, but the treasured new man in my life was already there waiting to surprise me with a gourmet bag lunch for my trip. It was a gesture so romantic that, as much as I was looking forward to the trip, I was sorry I was leaving. The following week I was back at Penn Station, this time off to a four-day writers conference.

Throughout these trips, we kept in touch through Skype and FaceTime chats, the conversations at a distance continuing to draw us closer. One of the more profound losses I experienced with Geoff's illness and death was the absence of an intimate, trusting relationship that provided reciprocal support and encouragement. As Geoff would put it, you want someone in your corner, who always has your back and keeps you pumped up—and I realized how much I longed to have that again in my life. As we slowly got to know each other better through those long-distance chats, that sort of bond developed between us, boosting my confidence and giving buoyancy to my outlook on the future.

The fact that we'd met so anonymously seemed to trouble close friends. But having expressed my feelings for a new man in my life, I left myself open to being quizzed and, worse, given unsolicited counsel. I was warned and told hoary tales meant to caution me about jumping into a relationship too quickly, making me, at this tender stage, defensive. *Would meeting him at a singles mixer or through an online dating service have provided greater guarantees?* I wondered. For the most part, I recognized that friends were cautioning me out of genuine care and concern. I was also aware that close pals were apprehensive about what sort of impact this new relationship might have on long-standing friendships. He was clearly the "un-Geoff" in so many ways; would he pull me away from my circle of friends?

My assurances on all fronts held little sway. As his toothbrush joined mine in a water glass and we began spending more time together, my own private thoughts on the matter came with a melody: que será, será. Whatever will be, will be.

Chapter Nineteen

If not now, when? meant fulfilling my wish list of adventurous places to visit, exciting things to do. At the top of that list was the most anticipated travel I'd booked that spring, a long-awaited trip to Havana, Cuba, in mid-May. I have wanted to go to Cuba since I was in high school—and nearly did when I was sixteen years old. I'd won a theatre scholarship to attend a summer program at Northwestern University in Evanston, Illinois, a full day's train ride from my home in Robbinsdale, Minnesota. Back then I considered a trip to Minneapolis exciting, but seeing Chicago for the first time was beyond thrilling. I was so blown away by the intense nine-week theatre program that when it ended I didn't want to go home to another year of high school. Boring! I was hungry for adventure. What I had in mind was Havana.

The newspapers were full of stories about the young revolutionary Fidel Castro, who'd overthrown the Batista regime. But being on the spot to witness the political upheaval was not what seduced me. I was reading Hemingway at the time. I knew about daiquiris at the Floridita. I'd pored over photographs in *Life* magazine of palm trees, white sands and azure seas. I imagined hot, languid Caribbean nights of decadence, glamour and intrigue. Cuba was a place of rum, bikinis, cigar smoke and dark, dangerous men. It was not something you could find in downtown Minneapolis, no matter how hard you looked. I ached to go.

I figured I had enough pocket money left for a bus ride to Miami, and from there I'd somehow make it to Havana where, of course, I'd find work harvesting sugarcane. I'd grown up on a farm, after all, and knew my way around a tractor. Unfortunately, my parents got wind of my hankerings. They piled into the family sedan and made it to Evanston in time for graduation. My father was none too pleased to be dragged off during harvest season to rescue his errant daughter. The next day, I sat in the back seat with my kid brother for the long ride home to Robbinsdale and my final year of high school.

Some fifty years later, as diplomatic relations between our two countries began to defrost, I was finally on my way to Cuba—if not now, when!

I traveled with a group of friends led by the president of the Beverly Hills Women's Club, Mumsey Nemiroff, an engaging art historian and lecturer. The trip was organized to coincide with the 12th Bienal de la Habana, a Havana gala exhibition inaugurated in 1984 to promote Latin American and Caribbean art.

Angela, a book-club friend I'd first met when we both served on the board of the Beverly Hills Women's Club, would be my room-mate on the trip. She was as impetuous as she was good hearted, so I knew sharing a room with Angela would be eventful. A year earlier she'd toured East Africa with Mumsey, choosing to dine on steak tar-tare the first night of the three-week trip—her consumption of raw meat practically guaranteeing the five-day confinement in a hospital that followed. However, she bonded with the doctor who got her well again and promptly began organizing a charity benefit for his clinic. American born but raised in her family's native Mexico, she was flu-ent in Spanish, which I figured would come in handy. The two of us spent our first night together in Miami drinking mojitos to acclimatize ourselves.

The following afternoon, we boarded a Gulfstream Air Charter for the hour-long flight from Miami to Jose Marti International Airport, where we deplaned the old-fashioned way, clambering down stairs and straggling across the breezy tarmac to Immigration Control. By late afternoon we'd checked into the Hotel NH Capri La Habana, one of Havana's most notorious casino-resort hotels, once owned and operated by racketeers, with actor George Raft serving as the legitimate front man. We unpacked in minutes and raced up to the famous rooftop pool for mojitos and an amazing view of the sea and city. Cuba!

When we returned to the Capri after dinner, I tried to Skype, but an Internet connection was available only with a prepaid card. The hotel had run out of them, and their telephone service had shut down. Angela managed to secure us a single card by charming someone at the front desk. I sent a hasty email: *Cuba is fantastic—and maddening! The air conditioning in our room doesn't work and it's a hundred degrees. Tried to call you but the switchboard could not get an outside line . . . Skype impossible! Crazy wonderful, a time warp fantasy . . . everyone just makes do . . . much talk of cigars here . . . will see what I can get for you tomorrow. Miss you!*

The following morning, I bought the cigars he wanted plus a few Cohibas that were recommended after a tour of the historic Partagás Cigar Factory. In a charming sepia-hued old building, we climbed creaky stairs to watch workers expertly hand roll tobacco leaves to create Cuba's most famous handmade export, the *Habanos* cigar—which Angela and I purchased in abundance as gifts, my one great splurge. Giggling like schoolgirls, we lit up and took turns puffing on one of our classy stogies, deeming it a one-time only experiment—if not in Cuba, when?

The primary aim of the Bienal de la Habana is to promote Cuban contemporary art, and to that end, the entire city was turned into a vast art gallery—art installations were everywhere. It was an awe-inspiring spectacle. Havana showed off its art and artists in restaurants, front gardens, backyards and rooftops, parks and the waterfront quay, artist's studios and galleries and even demolition sites and a former battle fortress. We toured the National Museum of Fine Arts Cuban Arts collection and attended the gala opening of the 12th Havana Biennial in the Wifredo Lam Centre of Contemporary Art, dedicated to Cuban surrealist painter Wifredo Lam, often referred to as the Cuban Picasso. But then Havana itself was a wondrous work of art: vivid, unexpected and enthralling.

Each day we managed to visit two or more artists in their studios, but if I were to single out an experience that encapsulates my thrall with Cuba and its artists, it would be an afternoon visit to a particularly dilapidated neighborhood in Havana and the home studio of Pedro Luis Cuéllar. The twenty-year-old sculptor works on small-scale pieces using found materials—wire, nuts, bolts, nails, string—to create delicate but powerful works of art that evoke the precariousness of life. The pieces are both darkly comic and frightening in their intensity, a reflection of the young man's personal family history and the tragic death of his father.

In this rundown neighborhood, the pin-neat, two-story house where Pedro lives with his mother and protective older brother gleams like a jewel in the dust, its handsome renovation made possible with the sale of only two pieces of his artwork. In Cuba, artists rank high among its most celebrated, prosperous inhabitants. Fine art is one of the country's greatest exports, and Angela did her part by purchasing one of Pedro Luis Cuéllar's fine sculptural pieces.

One of my fondest memories of the year I lived in Paris was an afternoon spent with James Jones, the celebrated author of *From Here to Eternity*, whose book *The Merry Month of May*, about the 1968 student revolt in Paris, had just been published. He was an avowed admirer of Hemingway, and after lunch, he took me on a walking tour of Hemingway haunts. As we strolled through the neighborhood where Hemingway had lived with his first wife, Hadley, Jones told me the struggling young writer had made ends meet by pawning items—but never his typewriter! At a pawnshop Hemingway was said to have frequented, Jones bought me an old bowler hat for a few francs, a keepsake I treasure to this day.

I was enchanted by the wonderful anecdotes Jones related, but more than anything, I was charmed that this acclaimed writer was so in awe of Ernest Hemingway that he'd made it his mission to seek out these places. Naturally, we ended our walk with an aperitif at one of Hemingway's favorite haunts, La Closerie des Lilas. It's not surprising, then, that during my weeklong trip to Cuba I would want to seek out Hemingway's Havana, a city he loved as much as its inhabitants revered the man known as "Papa."

I'm also a great fan of Hemingway, whose stories made me long to visit Havana when I was still in high school—and here was my chance to walk in his footsteps. My first stop was La Bodeguita del Medio on Empedrado Street, only a block away from the Plaza de la Catedral in Old Havana. I'd thought the daiquiri was Hemingway's cocktail of choice, but according to the La Bodeguita del Medio, he favored the mojito. The Cuban highball, made with crushed mint, lime juice, sugar and, of course, rum, may have originated at "La B del M," as it's known. Unfortunately, the bar wasn't open at 9:30 a.m. (not an unreasonable hour for a breakfast mojito) but I had a good peek inside before the gate was pulled shut.

Hotel Ambos Mundos, built in the 1920s near the Plaza de Armas, was the Hemingway site I was most eager to visit. It was here, in room 511, Hemingway's headquarters off and on between 1932 and 1939, that he began writing the opening chapters of *For Whom the Bell Tolls*. The fifth-floor corner room, with its shuttered French windows and charming view of rooftops and the nearby harbor, is enshrined, with framed photos and displays of memorabilia that include his typewriter, fishing rods, books, eyeglasses and the narrow bed tucked into an alcove. I stood for long minutes gazing at the copies of his books displayed in a glass-fronted cabinet, every title familiar to me. During my early years in London, I'd recorded many of Hemingway's short stories for BBC Radio.

Geoff was a great Hemingway fan, too, and I wished we could have visited room 511 together. We'd often attended the annual International Imitation Hemingway Competition dinner held in Harry's Bar & American Grill in Century City near the *Los Angeles* magazine offices. With that thought in mind, I imagined the old man himself looking up from his writing desk in the middle of the sun-filled room and scowling at us for enjoying those evenings of mock-Hemingway writing.

How much better if we could have enticed Hemingway to join us at perhaps the most iconic of his haunts, the El Floridita in Old Havana, where it's said he drank copious amounts of frozen daiquiris. Sadly, it was closed, which meant we couldn't engage in rivaling Hemingway's putative record of eleven cocktails by 11:00 a.m. But then, Angela and I were imbibing our share of mojitos and daiquiris elsewhere in Havana . . . and there's always next time.

Cuba is full of the sort of cars my dad hankered after when I was growing up, the luxurious, fin-tailed extravaganzas of the Eisenhower era.

They are now abundant only on the streets of Havana, time-stopped by the revolution in 1959, which cut off the free flow of Detroit-made Cadillacs and Oldsmobiles. Many of these magnificent relics now serve as taxis for awestruck tourists reminded of their own *American Graffiti* pasts.

One night after dinner, Mumsey arranged for us to tour the city in vintage Buick and Pontiac convertibles featuring gleaming chrome, bench seats and cosmic hood ornaments. Resplendent in glittering tropical hues of turquoise, hot pink, canary yellow and lipstick red, but lacking seat belts and air bags, these roomy land cruisers easily fit four in the back seat.

I slid in next to our driver, an amiable young Cuban with a gap-toothed smile, who steered one-handed. I suspected his other arm was busy holding the car door closed. It's only when you're inside one of these restored vehicles that you notice the patches of Bondo and miscellaneous wires dangling like spaghetti below the dashboards. I don't want to think about how many gallons per mile these glamorous babes consume, but even a cloud of exhaust fumes couldn't diminish the romance of gliding down boulevards in a vintage convertible under a starlit sky, a sultry breeze ruffling my hair.

But then, just as we were passing the decaying hulk of one of Meyer Lansky's once-elegant casino, my gallant driver turned snarly when a carload of wise guys jeered while trying to pass us on an inside lane. Our driver floored it, pedal to the metal, and I gulped a lungful of toxic fumes as we tore down the oceanfront boulevard in a drag race. I clutched the car door, which I discovered had no workable handle, my eyes trained on the sharp curve ahead. At the last, crucial moment, my driver veered into the right-hand lane, cutting off the fist-shaking roughnecks—and I survived to tell the tale.

Basking in the afterglow of our thrilling high-speed race, I gave my driver the kind of sidelong glance Natalie Wood would've given

James Dean. Then I wondered, was this staged for a carload of giggling *turistas*?

When we returned to the hotel, I walked the corridor outside our room in search of an elusive Internet signal—and found one! I quickly sent an email: *Cuba is magical . . . loving it . . . everything is an adventure, always unpredictable . . . went joyriding in a red-and-white vintage Buick, and the driver drag-raced another vehicle full of jeering kids . . . Only lasted a death-defying half minute—and I wouldn't have missed it.*

Angela and I decided the Internet cards were a scam, the advertised thirty minutes draining with a single quick email. She took a funny picture of me sitting on the floor at the far end of our hallway, a glass of wine within reach, still hoping to Skype. But then, the phone in our room rang, and we raced to answer it . . . a call from New York! How had he managed to get through? It took several tries, he said, "but I got your email about joyriding and had to call."

How I looked forward to traveling with him—and we were already making plans to do so. Sicily was on the list. So were Paris and London. We were each eager to acquaint the other with familiar haunts, making them ours with new memories to share. The great joy of traveling with someone is seeing a place with fresh eyes and appreciating it all the more.

On our walking tour of Old Havana the next day, we strolled the cobbled streets to the famous Four Plazas of Old Havana:

Plaza de la Catedral, where one of the oldest cathedrals in the Americas was founded on this square bounded by the former mansions of the Spanish nobles;

Plaza de Armas, which was once the parade grounds of the Spanish troops but is now filled with stalls of antiquarian booksellers;

Plaza de San Francisco de Asís, which faces the cruise ship and ferry terminal where weekend vacationers from Miami would drive their cars off the overnight ferry to enjoy a wild jaunt in Havana—the origin of Cuba's car culture;

And Plaza Vieja, which is reminiscent of the Piazza San Marco in Venice and was once Havana's open marketplace.

Along the way, one had only to turn a corner or look into an alleyway to discover art installations tucked everywhere in galleries, gardens and pop-up spaces. One of the most interesting exhibits was the Maqueta de la Habana, a scale model of the original historic city of Havana. Osmany Suárez, a young professor of art history and anthropology at the University of Havana, described the process of the restoration of Old Havana, including the role of UNESCO. We also toured the Museum of Santeria (Museo Municipal de Guanabacoa), learning about various Afro-Cuban religions.

After our long walking tour in Old Havana, Angela and I decided to have cocktails at the Hotel Nacional de Cuba, a grand old landmark built in 1930 and only a short stroll from our hotel. The magnificent art deco hotel overlooks the Malecón, a lengthy boardwalk along the ocean, and broad, rolling lawns shaded with palm trees. Before ordering mojitos in the garden, we spent a good hour in the salon looking at displays of the hotel's extraordinary history, which, of course, included photographs not only of Hemingway but also of every other imaginable film star and world-class celebrity. The Nacional was one of the resorts operated by Meyer Lansky up to the moment of the revolution in 1959. During the Cuban Missile Crisis, antiaircraft emplacements were installed on the grounds.

Mumsey also arranged for us to attend the Opera de la Calle, one of Havana's musical-theatre companies, and watch an afternoon rehearsal of Ballet Folklorico de Cuba, an ensemble that presents Afro-Cuban music and dance. On Saturday night we went to a rocking concert in the hottest nightspot in Havana, the Fábrica de Arte Cubano (FAC), an arts, fashion and music entertainment complex in the postindustrial setting of a former cooking-oil factory. We sat at a table in an outdoor lounge area, surrounded by a raucous, pulsing crowd of young Cubans enjoying the multimedia musical performance.

All of our meals throughout our trip were in *paladares*, privately owned and operated in-home restaurants, as opposed to restaurants owned and operated by the Cuban-government. The paladares are very strictly regulated and limited to no more than fifty seats, and equipment and food supplies must be purchased at government-controlled facilities. In some cases, to preserve the "in-home" requirement, a room or space is set aside with minimal furnishings of a bed, chair and table. While some of the more upmarket, sophisticated paladares were well-appointed and artfully designed, some were clearly carved out of existing residences and made do with mismatched tables, chairs, flatware and dishes, which added to the charm.

Very often Mumsey would arrange lunch in the homes of artists, such as Kadir López, whose works are historically inspired multimedia installations combining advertising artifacts from pre-revolutionary Cuba. Prior to lunch, López discussed his art and trends in the local contemporary art scene with Howard Farber, a well-established American collector of contemporary Cuban art.

One of the more upscale establishments was the Soviet-inspired paladar Nazdarovie, with a spectacular view overlooking Havana's Malecón. Mumsey had invited Monsignor Veceslav, the chargé d'affaires for the diplomatic mission of the papal nuncio to Cuba, to join us and speak about the role of the Catholic Church in Cuba; his boss, Pope Francis; and the recent reopening of diplomatic relations between the United States and Cuba. Angela spoke at length with the monsignor, who was surprisingly young, very open and friendly.

Geoff would have loved the Atelier, a classic art-filled paladar in a Spanish colonial building in Vedado. I thought of him the following day when we had lunch in the stunning StarBien Restaurante in a renovated art deco mansion, also in Vedado. La Guarida, probably Havana's most famous paladar, was decorated with antique furnishings and chandeliers and located in a century-old mansion, again an experience Geoff would have appreciated and that undoubtedly would have made it into his magazine's annual restaurant guide.

Dining at various paladares gave us an opportunity to experience various traditional, contemporary and fusion cuisines in many different Havana neighborhoods. We had dinner at Paladar HM7, a brand-new slow-cooking-style paladar with a spectacular view of the Havana seafront—and located across the street from Meyer Lansky's Hotel Habana Riviera, in its time the most modern casino resort in the world. We had great criollo cuisine at paladar La Fontana. We ate at El Aljibe, an outdoor thatch-roof restaurant in Miramar, a few minutes from downtown Havana. Their specialty, El Aljibe chicken, was a plate heaped with flavorful roast chicken, French fries, fried plantain, black beans and rice.

We even went on a tour outside Havana to visit the organic farm of the Restaurante Mediterráneo-Havana, where we dined in Vedado. There we learned about Cuban agriculture, but also about the difficulties and solutions for proprietors in supplying and managing high-end paladares.

That night, I got another surprise call from New York and had to whisper because Angela, who had carefully pointed out safe things to eat, was in bed, having experienced an attack of Castro's revenge. I kept our chat brief, and after nursing poor Angela, who was feeling very unwell, I slipped out into the hallway and managed to snag Internet access to send an email message. *Only Angela! She's been delightful through one misadventure after another. Last night we missed our ride back to the hotel and ended up hitchhiking in a souped-up vintage Pontiac she hailed. Because she speaks Spanish and is so appealing, we engage more with Cubans in the streets. Sunday morning, she chatted with a little boy dressed in an immaculate white suit for his first communion. The other day, the young professor was enthralled by her at lunch, and we got to hear his amazing personal story. He's not yet thirty but is in charge of restoration of Old Havana. These private conversations, translated by Angela, have enriched this whole incredible experience.*

I was astonished at how much we were able to pack in, including an unforgettable tour of the incredibly beautiful Cueva del Indio, home to the local indigenous Guanahatabey people, who archeologists believe used the caves as a graveyard and refuge during the Spanish conquest. We walked through the large grotto, discovered in 1920, then took the underground boat ride to view the marvelous limestone formations. Afterward, we stopped at a working tobacco plantation.

Possibly my favorite excursion was to the Finca Agroecologica El Paraiso in Viñales. Having grown up on a farm, I felt very much at home walking in the fields among the rows of well-tended vegetables, then dining on a superb lunch of organically grown food. The blue-and-white farmhouse, with open verandas, looked out over fields to a vast panorama of distant hills. The tables were set with blue-checkered cloths and bottles of rum to top up a delicious coconut-based herbal drink. The meal came in waves of hearty family-style servings of soup, side dishes and savory meat courses, including a whole roast suckling pig displayed and carved in the restaurant—an off-putting sight, at first. In keeping with the in-home paladar dining, the family-owned farmhouse restaurant has a single room with a bed, chair and simple furnishings, but little sign of genuine occupation.

The occasion when I missed Geoff most was our last evening in Havana, when we went to the famous Tropicana, a dazzling casino and cabaret that opened in 1939 on the grounds of the Villa Mina estate. Hemingway visited this hedonistic, jet-set playground, famous for its exotic showgirls wearing sequins, feathers and not much else, and its decadent rum-soaked partying. We had ringside seats for the glitzy, fast-paced show, but I was just as enthralled by the building's sweeping modernist architecture and the glamorous retro flavor of the historic nightclub, which Geoff would have appreciated, too. At the end of the show, I was caught by surprise when one of the exotic male dancers, wearing little more than a suggestion of modesty, jumped off the stage and started boogying with me, all caught on video by Angela. Geoff, who knew how much I love dancing, would have found it hilarious!

Chapter Twenty

My long-awaited trip proved to be a profound experience, all that I imagined it would be and so much more. It was a weeklong immersion in Cuban culture, history, art and food and included visits to a dozen artists' studios, dining in private-home paladares, a trip to an organic farm in the countryside, an evening at the exotic Tropicana nightclub, an exploration of a hidden Indian cave, a tour of a cigar factory, a whiz around town in vintage fin-tailed automobiles and, of course, a daiquiri at one of Hemingway's many haunts. But surely the most unlikely sight I witnessed was a modern-day drone careening around inside a magnificent cathedral, an "art installation" that was mesmerizing, if unintended.

Although a new man has entered my world, Geoff is never far from my thoughts, just as I'm sure Barbara figured in his mind after we were together. Photographs of my husband remain in place throughout the apartment, his name crops up in conversation and I feel his presence in all aspects of my daily life. I know that won't change. No matter what direction my life takes, I'll carry him with me whatever new road I travel.

Nearly two years later, the man I met in the hallway is still in my life, too, although he's since returned to Europe to work. We stay in close touch through Skype and email, and meet to travel together when we can. It's a treasured relationship, one that we keep to ourselves, and it provides the intimate companionship, support and romance I was ready to welcome back into my life.

Writing and acting are still my primary focus, but I'm also finding purpose and meaningful experiences through volunteer work with CurePSP, a nonprofit foundation focused on neurodegenerative diseases, including the one that claimed my husband's life. Through CurePSP I took support-group training and met Audrey, with whom I'm partnering to form a support group for people diagnosed with prime-of-life diseases and their caregivers. Audrey's husband passed away from PSP in 2015, and their story is an inspiration to me.

Her husband Jeff, a gifted jazz guitarist, began losing his eyesight at age fifty-five. In June 2011, only two weeks before he was going out on the road again, he went completely blind. At the time, he thought he had a long life ahead of him as a musician and would have to adjust to being blind.

Audrey and Jeff discussed cancelling the tour, knowing that under the circumstances, everyone would understand. But, as Audrey told him, "Cancelling now will set a precedent for future work. Do you want that?"

Their older son, Chris, who was eleven years old, told him, "It's okay, Dad, you always play guitar with your eyes closed anyway."

Jeff boarded the flight on his own to play in New Orleans, then went on to Los Angeles for Jazz Fest West. There he met Stevie Wonder, who sat in on the same session. Stevie's advice to him on living blind was "Gotta stay up . . . show your abilities, not disabilities." Jeff took it to heart and lived by it, determined not to let blindness curtail his career.

"Nothing stopped him," Audrey said. "On Mother's Day, he walked miles to buy me a bouquet of roses. 'You didn't have to do that,' I told him. 'Yes, I did,' he said. 'I have to do things on my own. Stevie does.'"

Jeff's illness grew worse, and it was clear he had some neurological impairment—perhaps in addition to his blindness or perhaps the cause of it. The disease, whatever it was, became a fifth member of the family, affecting all of them as it worsened on a daily basis. At nine years old, their younger son Matthew was leading Jeff across the street. Roles flipped, but everyone pulled together and dealt with the changes.

According to Audrey, "Jeff was very open about having people see him ill. We were always surrounded by family and friends. The kids had all their pals in, and everyone felt comfortable being around Jeff, even when he became very frail."

He was eventually diagnosed with PSP and died two months later on New Year's Day. "The night before, the house was full of people," Audrey said. "Everyone spent time with him, including the friends of our sons. The biggest torture for Jeff was leaving his children."

Shortly before he died, Matthew asked his father if he was scared.

"Sort of," Jeff told him. "There's the unknown, but I'll handle it."

They nodded in agreement, and Matthew said, "I think you'll be better off, Dad."

"No doubt about it," Jeff said.

"It's a very personal choice, but Jeff was clear that he wanted quality of life with his family and would let nature take its course," Audrey said. "That meant no feeding tubes or extraordinary measures. Seeing a DNR bracelet on Jeff's wrist upset the boys, but we talked about it. They understood. He'd accomplished such a lot in his life and made peace with himself."

There are many of us, like Audrey and me, who become involved in support groups first to help ourselves face the challenges of caregiving, then later to utilize our experiences to provide comfort and practical assistance to others. I feel tremendous empathy for people newly diagnosed who are attending a support group meeting for the first time. Geoff had recently been diagnosed when I showed up at my first meeting, led by a retired nurse whose husband was a doctor and had died from PSP. All I knew about the disease was what I'd been able to find on the Internet, and I was devastated. I did not handle that initial session at all well—in fact, I burst into tears.

A woman who had been a long-term caregiver for her husband took me aside and listened to me pour my heart out. Her calm, compassionate demeanor helped me to get a grip on my emotions and adopt a more practical, optimistic attitude that would benefit me in caring for Geoff. The woman set an example that I wanted to emulate after my husband passed away.

At a CurePSP family conference for caregivers, Audrey's words struck a chord with me and for everyone attending when she said: "I know each of our journeys is different, but in many ways they are the same. We share the common thread of endless hours of despair, exhaustion, fear, anger, hopelessness and heartbreak. This is a lonely journey without a roadmap to follow, and that's why we're all here to give each other support."

Over the past several years, I've been a volunteer speaker on behalf of CurePSP at various events and conferences across the country. I often choose as my theme "If Not Now, When?" because it offers a positive message, one that's hopeful and proactive in the face of chronic and terminal illness.

"If not now, when?" means something different for everyone I meet at these gatherings. For some it's ticking off bucket-list aspirations, but for most it's just aiming to enjoy meaningful time and make the most out of life each day with a loved one.

My friend Diane, who lives in New York and is a caregiver for her mother, proves that you don't have to travel far to visit exotic, soul-enriching sites. Diane, whose mother has advanced COPD, signed up for a special museum membership that gives them access to affordable day trips in the city. They visit the Museum of Modern Art, where they sit in the sculpture garden, and the Temple of Dendur at the Metropolitan Museum of Art, one of her mother's favorite places.

"She tires easily, but I can push her wheelchair through the botanical gardens and other venues that give both of us pleasure and time together."

My parents didn't wait for "someday," either. In 1946, anxious to be back with family in my father's war-torn homeland, they packed up three young children to travel over the Atlantic. Because my father still owned a farm there, our family was among the first wave of civilians permitted to travel by ship back to Norway, where we lived for a year.

After returning to live in Minnesota, my parents somehow managed, even on a modest farm-family's budget, to visit Norway every other year. Once my two brothers and I were on our own, the Virgin Islands, Hawaii and Alaska were on my parents' travel agenda. They continued their wide-ranging travels even when my father developed a neurological condition that necessitated using a walker and eventually a wheelchair. Little deterred them; the anticipation, the travel itself and the afterglow once they returned home made those trips worthwhile.

"Travel now, when you can," my mother always encouraged us. "You never know what's down the road."

Soon, I'll join my brothers and three generations of our extended family in a reunion celebration at the old homestead on the shores of a fjord in Northern Norway. On a very long summer day in late June, as the midnight sun glimmers behind the tips of mountains for the briefest moment before rising again, I'll be visiting with all the cousins I lived among and played with as a child.

Thinking of this reminds me of Jane's words to me the last time I saw her: "We come into this world alone and leave it alone; we must make peace with who we are and what we leave behind."

I realize I'm now approximately the same age Jane was when we first met in London. She was then living a solitary life, embracing new pursuits and experiences, and enjoying the company of a younger man in her life. She was also teaching, mentoring me in ways I appreciated at the time and value even more as I've gained perspective on those magical Wednesday afternoons with her. Perhaps I shouldn't be surprised at the many parallels in our lives, because we connected on an almost psychic level from the beginning. I have no doubt she was imparting valuable lessons back then that I would assimilate only later in my life. In my own way, I hope I'm passing along the life lessons she taught me.

I see certain elements of Jane in myself—not in her penchant for tea gowns and her pouf of lavender hair, but rather in the way she lived. I'd like to think I share her exuberance for life, her capacity to handle adversity and the manner in which she embraced each new life passage as it unfolded. If I were to sum her up in a fleeting glimpse, it would be a snapshot of Jane during our last tea together. Though frail and nearing her end, her eyes gleamed in joyous expectation as she raised a forkful of chocolate-mousse cake to her lips.

Before I face my own reckoning, there is still so much I want to experience in life. As Jane would have whispered in my ear, "If not now, when?"

ACKNOWLEDGMENTS

"If I am not for myself, who is for me? And when I am for myself, what am I? And if not now, when?" is a quote attributed to Hillel the Elder, a Jewish leader who lived in the first century. Variations on the quote have been used by, among many others, John F. Kennedy, Ronald Reagan, George W. Bush and Barack Obama as a call to assume responsibility and take action.

Decades ago when Jane, my teacher and mentor, first uttered the words "If not now, when?" to me, I understood her to mean, "get on with it, girl—it's time!" Over the years, the expression has become my own way of reminding myself to seize an opportunity and not count on an uncertain future. When I became my husband's caregiver and knew our time together was limited, "If not now, when?" took on far greater significance. I wanted to make the most of our days so I could carry those memories with me in a world without him.

My deepest thanks to all our devoted friends and family members for their tremendous support and encouragement. My gratitude to Amy Hosford for giving me the opportunity to share our story, to Andrew Pantoja for his excellent editorial guidance and to everyone at Grand Harbor for their care and dedication. As always, my great thanks to Cynthia Manson, my agent, for her superb representation, and to Caitlin Alexander, a wonderful editor who has taught me so much and always makes me look good.

ABOUT THE AUTHOR

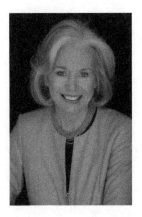

Kathryn Leigh Scott is an author, actress, and a volunteer spokesperson for the national CurePSP foundation. She grew up on a farm in Robbinsdale, Minnesota, and resides in New York City and Los Angeles.